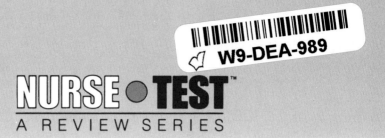

MEDICAL-SURGICAL NURSING

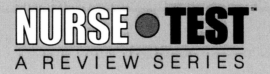

MEDICAL-SURGICAL NURSING

Frances L. Martin, RN,C, MSN, MSEd
Assistant Professor of Nursing
College of Staten Island
Staten Island, N.Y.

Series Editor
Laura Gasparis Vonfrolio, RN, MA, CCRN, CEN
Assistant Professor of Nursing
College of Staten Island
Staten Island, N.Y.

Springhouse Corporation
Springhouse, Pennsylvania

Staff

Executive Director, Editorial
Stanley Loeb

Director of Trade and Textbooks
Minnie B. Rose, RN, BSN, MEd

Art Director
John Hubbard

Clinical Consultant
Maryann Foley, RN, BSN

Editors
Diane Labus, Keith de Pinho

Copy Editors
Traci A. Ginnona, Mary Hohenhaus Hardy, Elizabeth Kiselev

Designers
Stephanie Peters (associate art director), Julie Carleton Barlow

Cover Illustration
Marianne Hughes

Manufacturing
Deborah Meiris (manager), T.A. Landis, Jennifer Suter

Printed in the United States of America.
NTQA3-041293

Library of Congress Cataloging-in-Publication Data

Martin, Frances L.
  Medical-surgical nursing/Frances·L. Martin.
    p. cm.—(NurseTest)
    Includes bibliographical references and index.
    1. Nursing—Examinations, questions, etc. 2. Surgical nursing—Examinations, questions, etc. I. Title. II. Series.
    [DNLM: 1. Nursing Care—examination questions. 2. Surgical Nursing—examination questions. WY 18 M379m]
RT55.M26 1992
610.73 076—dc20
DNLM/DLC   91-4836
ISBN 0-87434-303-8   CIP

Contents

Consultant and Contributors

Consultant

Sondra G. Ferguson, RN, MSN, CS, CCRN, Clinical Specialist for Critical Care, Veterans' Affairs Medical Center, Lexington, Ky.

Contributors

Iqbal A. Ansari, MD, FACA, FCCP, Attending Anesthesiologist, Methodist Hospital, Brooklyn, N.Y.

Susan Apold-Giampietro, RN, MSN, Substitute Instructor, Lehman College, Bronx, N.Y.

Carmelle Bellefleur, RN, MSN, Assistant Professor, New York City Technical College, Brooklyn, N.Y.

Donna M. Bellovics, RN, EdD, Associate Professor and Chairperson, Department of Nursing, Cameron University, Lawton, Okla.

Lorraine Boykin, RD, EdD, Professor Emeritus, Hunter College, New York.

Mary T. Boylston, RN, MSN, CCRN, Instructor, Eastern College, St. Davids, Pa.

Glenna L. Carter, RN, MSN, Professor of Nursing (retired), Vincennes (Ind.) University.

Claudia Christman, RN,C, BSN, MS, CPT, AN, Assistant Director, Nurse Practitioner, Adult Course, Silas B. Hayes Army Community Hospital, Fort Ord, Calif.

Margaret A. Cunningham, RN, MS, CDE, Diabetes Clinical Nurse Specialist, Loyola University, Mulcahy Outpatient Center, Maywood, Ill.

Eileen Greif Fishbein, RN, DNSc, Assistant Professor, Georgetown University, Washington, D.C.

Sarah A. Ghent, RN, AAS, Former Case Management Coordinator, Health Insurance Plan of Greater New York.

Linda M. Goodfellow, RN, MNEd, Nurse Educator and Private Consultant, Pittsburgh.

Alice Geraghty Graham, RN, BSN, MA, MS, Assistant Professor of Nursing, College of Staten Island, N.Y.

Ann Harley, RN, EdD, Assistant Dean for Academic Affairs, Bellin College of Nursing, Green Bay, Wis.

Marlene Bullock Harvey, RN, MEd, Assistant Professor, Long Island University, Brooklyn, N.Y.

Milagros Ilea, RN, MA, Former Assistant Professor, Lienhard School of Nursing, Pace University, New York.

Mary Pat Casey Lynch, RN, BSN, CCRN, Assistant Head Nurse (ICU), Pennsylvania Hospital, Philadelphia.

Frances L. Martin, RN,C, MSN, MSE, Assistant Professor of Nursing, College of Staten Island, N.Y.

Ruth Ann Miller, RN, BSN, Staff Nurse (MICU), St. Anthony Medical Center, Columbus, Ohio

Karen McGough Monks, RN, MSN, Division Chairman of Human Sciences, Arizona Western College, Yuma.

Barbara A. Moyer, RN, MSN, Assistant Professor, Allentown College of St. Francis de Sales, Center Valley, Pa.; Clinical Educator, Lehigh Valley Hospital Center, Allentown, Pa.

Geri Budeshein Neuberger, RN, MN, EdD, Associate Professor, University of Kansas, School of Nursing, Kansas City.

Pearline Okumakpeyi, RN, BSN, MA, Assistant Professor, New York City Technical College, Brooklyn, N.Y.

Lois J. Owen, RN, PhD, Associate Professor, Cleveland State University, Cleveland, Ohio

Thena E. Parrott, RN, MS, Faculty, Central Texas College, American Education Complex, Killeen.

Holly J. Price, RN, MSN, Clinical Specialist in Gerontology, Instructor, Providence Hospital School of Nursing, Sandusky, Ohio

Barbara Quattlebaum, RN, MS, Assistant Administrator, Waterview Nursing Care Center, New York.

Barbara Ann Russo, RN, MA, MEd, Associate Professor, Hunter College, New York.

Francis Scelsi, RN, Former Health Service Supervisor, Golden Gate Health Care Center, Staten Island, N.Y.

Mary Beth Tedesco, RN, BSN, MNEd, CRRN, Nursing Coordinator, Harmarville Rehabilitation Center, Pittsburgh.

Laura Gasparis Vonfrolio, RN, MA, CCRN, CEN, Assistant Professor of Nursing, College of Staten Island, N.Y.

Jane C. Walton, RN, MS, Assistant Unit Leader, Johnston R. Bowman Health Care Center for the Elderly, Rush-Presbyterian-St. Luke's Medical Center, Chicago.

Acknowledgments and Dedication

This book would not have become a reality without the commitment and support of many individuals. I give special thanks to my colleague, Laura Gasparis Vonfrolio, who initiated this project. Laura constantly encouraged me and provided feedback during the many months of research, writing, and rewriting. Also, I would like to commend the typists—Fay Gasparis, Mary Geisler, Tina Quilty, and Amelia Granelli. They did a phenomenal job of deciphering volumes of written material, which was not always very legible, under a tight schedule.

In memory of my mother, Mrs. Nellie Marshall,
and in honor of my daughter, Tanya.

Preface

This book is one in a series designed to help nursing students, professional licensed or registered nurses, nurses educated abroad, and nurses returning to the field improve their test-taking skills and increase their theoretical knowledge of nursing. It features case-study situations and a multiple-choice question-and-answer format similar to that used in NCLEX-RN (National Council Licensure Examination for Registered Nurses) and nursing challenge examinations. It also includes a comprehensive examination to test overall knowledge of questions and answers presented in each of the chapters. *Medical-Surgical Nursing,* which offers questions about theoretical and clinical information covered in most basic medical-surgical textbooks, is arranged by body system. Topics focus on:

- identifying pertinent assessment data for selected disorders
- interpreting diagnostic tests
- assigning appropriate nursing diagnoses
- prioritizing nursing interventions
- developing patient care plans
- building communication skills
- carrying out patient treatments, such as drug therapy
- preventing treatment complications
- providing patient teaching.

When using this book, remember to begin with the first question in each chapter and proceed in a sequential manner. Do not skip around, because subsequent answers may build on previous ones.

Introduction

Nurses are tested continually throughout their careers—as nursing students in the classroom, as professionals undergoing licensure or certification, and as practicing clinicians in the health care field. Such testing helps to measure acquired knowledge and ultimately prepares nurses for real-life clinical situations.

Because testing knowledge is an important, ongoing aspect of a nurse's career and heavy emphasis is placed upon passing certain critical examinations, such as NCLEX-RN (National Council Licensure Examination for Registered Nurses) and nursing challenge examinations, nurses must rely on practical study guides and effective test-taking strategies if they are to succeed.

NurseTest: A Review Series was developed to help nurses improve their test-taking abilities and increase their general clinical knowledge. Each book in the series focuses on a specific area of study or a speciality of nursing practice. Written in a question-and-answer format, each book includes hundreds of questions built on case-study situations and a final comprehensive examination that tests overall subject knowledge. All questions, which appear at the beginning of each chapter, include four possible answers. The correct answers—along with rationales explaining why the correct answers are appropriate choices and why the incorrect answers are inappropriate—appear at the end of each chapter. A blank answer sheet is provided in each chapter.

Although having a thorough understanding of the clinical material is probably the best way to ensure good test results, developing and implementing good test-taking strategies may mean the difference between passing and failing. Such strategies include physical and mental preparation, paying attention to directions, keeping track of the time, and reading the questions and answer choices carefully to determine the most appropriate response.

Preparing for the test

Regardless of your reason for taking the test, you'll need to be prepared. If you are like many nurses, this may mean extensive reading, note taking, studying, and reviewing. Therefore, developing good study habits is vital. Whether studying alone or in a group, you'll do well to follow a few simple rules:
- Find a place that is conducive to studying, such as a library, study hall, or lounge, if distractions are a problem.
- Limit your studying to several short sessions rather than one long cramming session.
- Highlight only the most essential information, and take selective notes.
- Concentrate on the most difficult or least familiar information first, saving the most familiar information for last.

Anticipate feeling some anxiety over the test, but try to find ways to relieve it. For example, try practicing deep-breathing exercises and other forms of relaxation, such as rhythmically tensing and relaxing muscle groups throughout your body. Practicing such exercises the night before the test and even while the papers are being distributed alleviates tension and promotes better concentration.

After what seems like countless hours of studying for an important test, the most effective final preparation is to relax and take it easy. Last-minute cramming can do little to increase knowledge and may cause unneeded stress and fatigue

Exercising or going to a movie the night before the test—then getting a good night's sleep—is usually most helpful.

Taking the test
Before answering any questions, remember to focus on the cardinal rules of test taking:
- Pay attention to directions.
- Read all instructions and questions carefully.
- Answer only what is being asked; do not read into a question anything beyond what is there.
- Know how much time is allotted for the test, and pace yourself accordingly. Be sure to note the halfway time.
- Scan the first page for a question you can answer easily, and mark the answer in the appropriate space on the answer sheet. Then go back to the first question and begin answering the questions in consecutive order. Answering an easy question first may give you a boost of confidence.
- Do not spend excessive time on any one question. If a question seems too difficult or complex, skip the question but remember to circle the number on the answer sheet; then return to the question after completing the other questions.
- Never leave an answer blank or mark two choices for the same answer.
- Compare the test to the answer sheet periodically to ensure that you haven't made any slight but costly errors, such as answering question 4 in question 5's space on the answer sheet.
- Erase all stray marks from the answer sheet before handing in the test.

Choosing the correct response
In a multiple-choice test, determining the correct answer to a question can sometimes be difficult. However, in many cases, you can successfully determine the correct answer by using one or more of the strategies listed below:
- Eliminate any obviously incorrect choices; then, reevaluate the remaining options and choose the most likely response. Ideally, you should try to narrow your choices to two likely options, affording yourself a 50% chance of choosing the correct answer. If choosing between the two remaining options seems especially difficult, take an educated guess.

- Look for key words or phrases in the question that can point to a correct response. For example, questions including the words "best," "most appropriate," or "most accurate" usually suggest that the correct response is a true statement, whereas those including "all...except," "least effective," and "least appropriate" usually suggest a false statement as the correct response. Such key words as "immediately," "promptly," and "highest priority" usually indicate that the correct response is something a nurse would normally do first.
- Look for interlocking clues, in which the correct response to one question forms the basis of the next question:

---

1 The nurse is caring for Mr. P., who is exhibiting abnormal extension and adduction of the arms, pronation of the wrists, and flexion of the fingers. Which type of posturing is characterized by such abnormalities?
A. Decorticate
B. Apraxic
C. Akinetic
D. Decerebrate

---

2 The nurse explains to Mr. P.'s daughter that decerebrate posturing typically results from:
A. Temporary lack of oxygen to the brain
B. Infection
C. Brain stem damage
D. Extrapyramidal system damage

In this example, "decerebrate" (the focus of the second question) is the correct answer to the first question. Although the mere repetition of "decerebrate" might suggest that it is the correct response, the real interlocking clue lies in the logical transition from one question to the other: in this case, the nurse cares for a patient exhibiting abnormal posturing, then explains the nature of such posturing to the patient's daughter.

Important: When looking for interlocking clues, always remember to read the questions and answer choices carefully, as choosing an answer solely on the basis of its repetition in another question can sometimes backfire:

1 Which type of posturing is characterized by abnormal flexion and adduction of the arms and by flexion of the fingers and wrists on the chest?
A. Decorticate
B. Apraxic
C. Akinetic
D. Decerebrate

2 The nurse understands that decerebrate posturing typically results from:
A. Temporary lack of oxygen to the brain
B. Infection
C. Brain stem damage
D. Extrapyramidal system damage

In this second example, "decerebrate" appears as an answer choice in the first question as well as the focus of the second question. Despite its repetition, however, "decerebrate" is not the correct response to the first question ("decorticate" is correct). The two questions are independent of each other, and no logical transition (or interlocking clue) exists.

After the test
Once you have completed the test, try to put it out of your mind; nothing can change the outcome at this point. Later, however, take time to review the test, if you're given an opportunity to do so—reviewing the questions and answers may provide some insight for future experiences. Otherwise, be satisfied with your accomplishment, and resume your usual work and leisure activities while you wait for the results. And expect to be pleasantly surprised.

Alice Geraghty Graham, RN, BSN, MA, MS
Assistant Professor of Nursing
College of Staten Island
Staten Island, N.Y.

CHAPTER 1

Respiratory System

Questions

1 Mr. R., a patient with patchy pneumonitis and atelectasis, experiences acute respiratory failure. The partial pressure of oxygen in arterial blood (PaO_2) at room air is 55 mm Hg. The most likely cause of hypoxemia in Mr. R. is:

A. Mechanical deposits
B. Anatomic dead space
C. Capillary shunting and shunt effect
D. Oxygen diffusion defect

2 Which type of surgery is most likely to predispose a patient to postoperative atelectasis, pneumonitis, or respiratory failure?

A. Upper abdominal surgery on an obese patient with a long history of smoking
B. Upper abdominal surgery on a patient with normal pulmonary function
C. Lower abdominal surgery on a young patient with diabetes mellitus
D. Surgery on the extremities of a nonsmoking football player

3 The most significant pulmonary change in a patient after upper abdominal surgery would be:

A. Altered respiratory rate
B. Increased tidal volume
C. Decreased vital capacity
D. Increased lung compliance

4 The primary reason for establishing an artificial airway in a patient is to:

A. Stimulate coughing
B. Facilitate postural drainage
C. Remove secretions and provide ventilation
D. Increase vital capacity

5 Mr. G., a patient with status asthmaticus, becomes less responsive. Arterial blood gas analysis reveals a partial pressure of carbon dioxide in arterial blood ($PaCO_2$) of 60 mm Hg and a PaO_2 of 50 mm Hg. The data most likely indicate acute:

A. Pulmonary embolism
B. Pulmonary edema
C. Respiratory failure
D. Pneumonitis

6 Mr. F., a patient on a volume-cycled ventilator, has a PaO_2 of 45 mm Hg on 40% inspired oxygen and a pH and a $PaCO_2$ within acceptable ranges. The nurse should:

A. Increase the respiratory rate
B. Increase the tidal volume
C. Increase the driving pressure
D. Initiate positive end-expiratory pressure therapy

SITUATION

Mr. E., age 38, is referred to the local hospital clinic after he has a positive tuberculin skin test result. He is admitted for further diagnostic evaluation. His orders include 300 mg of isoniazid (Laniazid) P.O. daily, 600 mg of rifampin (Rimactane) P.O. daily, 100 mg of pyridoxine (vitamin B6) P.O. daily, regular diet, and bed rest.

Questions 7 to 13 refer to this situation.

---

7 Which would most likely confirm Mr. E.'s diagnosis of tuberculosis (TB)?

A. Creatine kinase (CK) test
B. Chest X-ray
C. Sputum smear and culture
D. White blood cell count

---

8 Which clinical manifestations would the nurse expect in a patient with TB?

A. Hemoptysis and weight gain
B. Dry cough and blood-streaked sputum
C. Productive cough and afternoon elevated temperature
D. Night sweats and urticaria

---

9 The TB diagnosis is confirmed, and Mr. E. is put on respiratory isolation. Mr. E. asks why this is necessary. The nurse should explain that:

A. TB is like other respiratory infections
B. TB is transmitted via inhalation of droplets containing diseased nuclei
C. Persons who have been exposed to TB are sensitized
D. Close contact is necessary for TB transmission

10 When providing care for Mr. E. during his isolation period, the nurse must *always* wear:

A. Rubber gloves
B. A face mask
C. An isolation gown
D. Isolation booties

11 Which nursing activity would be most therapeutic while Mr. E. is on bed rest?

A. Encouraging family and friends to visit him three times a day
B. Assisting him in walking to the lounge
C. Assisting him with range-of-motion exercises
D. Encouraging him to visit other patients

12 Possible adverse effects of isoniazid therapy include:

A. Peripheral neuritis, tachycardia, and insomnia
B. Fever and GI dysfunction
C. Hepatic dysfunction, headache, and vertigo
D. Hepatic dysfunction and kidney damage

13 After a week in the hospital, Mr. E. is ready for discharge. When providing discharge instructions, the nurse should discuss all of the following topics *except:*

A. The plan for regular follow-up care
B. The possible adverse effects of his medications
C. The need to discontinue isoniazid if nausea occurs
D. The need to cover his nose and mouth with disposable tissues when coughing, sneezing, and laughing

---

SITUATION

Mr. M., a 53-year-old mine worker, is admitted to the hospital after his physician detects a lesion on his chest X-ray during an annual physical examination. A lung biopsy confirms a diagnosis of sarcoidosis.

Questions 14 to 16 refer to this situation.

14 Sarcoidosis is best defined as:

A. An occupational disease caused by air pollution
B. A disease characterized by multiple masses (granulomas) in most of the body's organs
C. A contagious disease that affects mostly blacks
D. A highly infectious disease of the respiratory tract

15 The physician orders 15 mg of prednisone (Deltasone) P.O. daily. To assess Mr. M. for adverse effects of this corticosteroid, the nurse should do all of the following *except:*

A. Observe for signs of hypoglycemia
B. Check blood glucose levels by fingerstick before meals and at bedtime
C. Weigh the patient daily
D. Observe for mood swings

16 To ensure that Mr. M. self-administers the corticosteroid properly, the nurse should give him all of the following discharge instructions *except:*

A. "Never abruptly discontinue the medication"
B. "Take the medication with food"
C. "Protect yourself against infection"
D. "Increase your salt intake"

SITUATION

N., a 19-year-old college student, is on the varsity football team. During a game, he is tackled and sustains fractured ribs on the right side of the chest. He is taken to the emergency department of a local hospital.

Questions 17 to 25 refer to this situation.

17 Which initial clinical manifestation should the nurse expect with this patient?

A. Paradoxical respiration
B. Shallow, painful breathing
C. Diminished breath sounds on the affected side
D. A clicking sensation during inspiration

18 N. becomes increasingly irritable and short of breath. A chest X-ray shows 30% of his right lung has collapsed. The patient receives oxygen via nasal cannula while awaiting chest tube insertion. At this point, the nurse should assess for which early sign of hypoxia?

A. Bradycardia
B. Restlessness
C. Low blood pressure
D. Glycosuria

19 N. asks the nurse, "What if I stop breathing completely when the physician inserts the chest tubes?" The most appropriate response would be to:

A. Explain what the tubes will do
B. Assure him that the nurse and physician will be present
C. Notify the physician to postpone the procedure
D. Ask a priest to talk with the patient before the procedure

20 The physician orders 5 mg of diazepam (Valium) I.V. before chest tube insertion primarily to:

A. Alleviate pain
B. Increase respiratory rate
C. Relieve anxiety and tension
D. Increase muscle activity

21 The physician inserts the chest tubes and attaches them to a water-seal drainage device set at 20 cm of suction. Then the physican orders a chest X-ray to:

A. Ascertain the position of the tubes
B. Advance the tubes 1 cm further
C. Visualize a single layer of the lungs
D. Record sound waves that penetrate the lungs

22 While N. is connected to the drainage device, the nurse should immediately report:

A. Excessive bubbling in the water-seal chamber
B. Fluctuation of fluid in the water-seal chamber
C. Dark red drainage in the collection chamber
D. A fluid level of 20 cm in the suction control chamber

23 To promote pulmonary ventilation, the nurse should include all of the following in this patient's care plan *except:*

A. Encouraging coughing and deep breathing
B. Providing hydration
C. Positioning the patient on his right side
D. Encouraging use of an incentive spirometer

24 Which observation would most likely indicate that N.'s chest tubes should be removed?

A. 120 ml of chest tube drainage in 24 hours
B. Cessation of pain and dyspnea
C. Absence of fluid fluctuation in the water-seal chamber
D. Lung reexpansion on chest X-ray

25 Which method would best prevent air from entering the pleural cavity after removal of N.'s chest tubes?

A. Breathing through pursed lips
B. Breathing quickly and shallowly (panting)
C. Breathing with an open mouth
D. Performing Valsalva's maneuver

SITUATION

Mr. B. has had a persistent cough for about 4 months. One week ago, he noted blood in his sputum. He is admitted to the hospital for diagnostic testing. The physician orders a bronchoscopy.

Questions 26 to 30 refer to this situation.

26 Immediately after the bronchoscopy, the nurse should withhold food and fluid until Mr. B.'s gag reflex returns, to prevent:

A. Aspiration
B. Abdominal distention
C. Dyspnea
D. Dyspepsia

27 Mr. B. is diagnosed with lung cancer. The physician orders various pulmonary function tests, including measurements of forced vital capacity and forced expiratory volume. The test results are used before surgery to:

A. Evaluate the spread of disease
B. Estimate the amount of anesthesia needed for surgery
C. Determine the amount of lung tissue to be removed
D. Calculate whether the contemplated surgery will leave enough functioning lung tissue

28 After a lobectomy, Mr. B. is returned to the unit with chest tubes in place. The nurse assigns a nursing diagnosis of *Impaired gas exchange related to lung alterations after surgery.* With this diagnosis, the expected outcome is that the patient will:

A. Report less chest pain
B. Assume a semi-Fowler's position
C. Request pain medication frequently
D. Exhibit a respiratory rate of less than 20 breaths/minute without dyspnea

29 Mr. B. will undergo radiation therapy on an outpatient basis to treat the cancer. When teaching Mr. B. about skin care, the nurse should encourage him to:

A. Use skin lotions and powders on the irradiated area
B. Avoid washing off the marks placed on his skin to guide radiation therapy
C. Wear constrictive clothing
D. Massage the irradiated area to increase circulation

30 Mr. B.'s wife is concerned about his poor appetite and weight loss. The nurse explains to her that radiation treatment, anxiety, and the disease itself can cause anorexia in cancer patients. The nurse should encourage Mr. B. to:

A. Limit activity before and after meals
B. Force fluids
C. Eat high-calorie foods
D. Eat hot meat dishes with special sauces

SITUATION

Mr. J., a 65-year-old retired steel mill worker, is admitted to the unit with dyspnea upon exertion. He has a long history of smoking. Initial assessment findings include barrel chest, ankle edema, persistent cough with copious sputum production, and variable wheezing on expiration. Laboratory test results include a hematocrit greater than 60% and a partial pressure of carbon dioxide in arterial blood (PaCO₂) of 65 mm Hg. The physician diagnoses chronic obstructive pulmonary disease (COPD).

Questions 31 to 37 refer to this situation.

31 Mr. J.'s ankle edema and respiratory problems should make the nurse suspect hypertrophy of which heart chamber?

A. Left atrium
B. Right atrium
C. Left ventricle
D. Right ventricle

32 The physician prescribes oxygen at 2 liters/minute via nasal cannula. Which statement best describes why Mr. J.'s oxygen therapy is maintained at this relatively low level?

A. Prolonged exposure to a high-oxygen environment causes structural damage to lung tissue
B. Increased oxygen concentrations of inspired air can cause alveoli to collapse
C. Oxygen therapy can eliminate the stimulus for breathing in a patient with chronic lung disease
D. Oxygen therapy may affect the eyes, causing tearing, edema, and visual impairment

33 The physician orders an aminophylline (Aminophyllin) I.V. drip for Mr. J. The nurse should be alert for which sign of drug toxicity?

A. Depression
B. Tachycardia
C. Lethargy
D. Cyanosis

34 Aterial blood gas (ABG) measurements reveal a pH of 7.25, a PaCO₂ of 62 mm Hg, and an HCO_3^- level of 22 mEq/liter. These results indicate:

A. Respiratory alkalosis
B. Respiratory acidosis
C. Metabolic alkalosis
D. Metabolic acidosis

35 During the nurse's morning rounds, she auscultates Mr. J.'s lungs and finds bilateral congestion and variable wheezing on expiration. The most appropriate nursing intervention would be to:

A. Take vital signs
B. Call the physician
C. Offer a cup of hot tea
D. Check heart sounds

36 Mr. J. is unable to exhale efficiently and becomes short of breath. The best nursing intervention would be to teach him:

A. Pursed-lip breathing
B. Coughing technique
C. Postural drainage
D. Relaxation techniques

37 The physician orders postural drainage for Mr. J. Which statement about postural drainage is most accurate?

A. Postural drainage uses gravity to augment mucociliary cleaning mechanisms and drain retained secretions
B. All patients with COPD are positioned the same way for postural drainage
C. Postural drainage involves rhythmic clapping of the chest wall with cupped hands
D. Postural drainage is effective only when performed for 1 hour or longer

---

SITUATION

A community health nurse visits Mr. Z., a 65-year-old diabetic patient, to review his diet and ability to self-administer insulin. During the visit, the nurse notes that Mr. Z.'s wife has a bad cough. After completing the visit with Mr. Z., the nurse speaks with Mrs. Z., who reports that she had shaking chills before the coughing started. She currently has difficulty breathing and pain in the right side of her chest. After consulting with Mrs. Z.'s physician, the nurse advises Mr. Z. to take his wife to the hospital for admission.

Questions 38 to 47 refer to this situation.

38 On admission, Mrs. Z. appears cyanotic. The cyanosis most likely is caused by:

A. Altered comfort
B. Iron deficiency anemia
C. Altered cardiac status
D. Impaired gas exchange

39 Because Mrs. Z. has dyspnea and is cyanotic, the nurse should observe her frequently for signs of cerebral hypoxia, including:

A. Irritability
B. Hyperactivity
C. Mental alertness
D. Frequent urination

40 The nurse evaluates Mrs. Z.'s cough and difficulty breathing through the mouth and decides the best route for obtaining a temperature reading would be:

A. Oral
B. Rectal
C. Axillary
D. Any of the above

41 Mrs. Z.'s physician orders an antitussive medication containing codeine. The purpose of the codeine is to:

A. Suppress the gag reflex
B. Decrease the frequency and intensity of coughing
C. Decrease irritation of the tracheal mucosa
D. Decrease chest pain

42 Which nursing intervention would most likely help loosen Mrs. Z.'s thick, tenacious respiratory secretions?

A. Performing postural drainage twice a day
B. Having her breathe humidified air
C. Telling her to cough and deep breathe every hour
D. Increasing her milk intake

43 The physician orders a sputum culture for Mrs. Z. When telling Mrs. Z. how to collect a sputum specimen, the nurse should include all of the following instructions *except:*

A. "Clear the nose and throat initially"
B. "Spit saliva and surface mucus into the sterile container"
C. "Take a few deep breaths before coughing"
D. "Use diaphragmatic contractions to help expel sputum"

44 The best time to collect a sputum specimen is:

A. Before bedtime
B. Midafternoon
C. Early in the morning
D. Any time during the day

45 The physician suspects that Mrs. Z. has bacterial pneumonia. The nurse would expect her sputum to be:

A. Bright red
B. Pink tinged
C. Rust colored
D. Thin and mucoid

46 The most common causative organism of bacterial pneumonia is:

A. *Streptococcus pneumoniae*
B. *Proteus*
C. *Haemophilus influenzae*
D. *Escherichia coli*

47 During a patient-teaching session on ways to prevent pneumonia, the nurse learns that Mrs. Z. has never been immunized against influenza. Before proceeding with her discussion of immunization, the nurse should determine if Mrs. Z. is allergic to:

A. Pollen
B. Cat dander
C. Eggs
D. Penicillin

SITUATION

Mrs. B., a patient with chronic emphysema, is admitted to the unit with acute respiratory failure. Endotracheal intubation and mechanical ventilation with high peak respiratory pressures are indicated. A chest X-ray shows multiple bullae. She suddenly develops tachypnea, tachycardia, and hypotension. Her chest is hyperresonant to percussion; auscultation reveals distant breath sounds. The physician diagnoses pneumothorax.

Questions 48 to 51 refer to this situation.

48 Which nursing action is the highest priority for this patient?

A. Scheduling her for an emergency perfusion scan
B. Preparing her for chest tube insertion
C. Initiating positive end-expiratory pressure therapy
D. Performing an electrocardiogram (ECG) immediately

49 Disconnecting the ventilator and vigorously suctioning Mrs. B. for a prolonged period could lead to all of the following complications *except:*

A. Hypoxemia
B. Cardiac arrhythmia
C. Hypotension
D. Septicemia

50 Which physiologic parameter indicates that weaning Mrs. B. from the ventilator is feasible?

A. Negative peak inspiratory pressure greater than -20 cm H_2O
B. Vital capacity of less than 10 ml/kg of body weight
C. PaO_2 of 100 mm Hg on 100% oxygen
D. Increase in shunt fraction

51 Before Mrs. B is weaned from the ventilator, all of the following conditions must be improved *except:*

A. Acid-base and electrolyte abnormalities
B. Caloric depletion
C. Infection
D. Anxiety

SITUATION

Mrs. J., age 45, is admitted to the unit with obesity hypoventilation syndrome (also called pickwickian syndrome). She is slightly dyspneic, hypotensive, and diaphoretic and complains of chronic fatigue, headaches, forgetfulness, and auditory hallucinations. Her husband states that she has difficulty sleeping at night, takes frequent daytime naps, and usually snores. She is 5 feet tall and weighs 300 lb. Her initial orders include a complete blood count immediately, ABG levels on room air, 500 mg of aminophylline in 500 ml of dextrose 5% in water at 20 ml/hour, and no sedatives.

Questions 52 to 55 refer to this situation.

52 After the aminophylline drip is started, Mrs. J's breathing pattern improves. This occurs because aminophylline:

A. Allows more air to enter the lungs
B. Decreases respiratory rate and depth
C. Helps the patient cough up thick secretions
D. Increases respiratory rate and depth

53 The nurse should assess Mrs. J. frequently for any adverse effects associated with aminophylline, including:

A. Abdominal pain, nausea, vomiting, and diarrhea
B. Hypotension, bradycardia, and mental depression
C. Headache, tachycardia, palpitations, and marked restlessness
D. Blurred vision, photophobia, and mydriasis

54 Which nursing assessment is the highest priority for Mrs. J.?

A. Respiratory assessment, noting rate, depth, and pattern of breathing
B. Nutritional assessment, focusing on dietary intake
C. Cardiovascular assessment, noting vital signs, pulses, and edema
D. Neurovascular assessment, noting orientation, extremity strength, and movement

55 Mrs. J. cannot sleep and requests a sedative. Based on the initial orders, the nurse's best response would be:

A. "You can't have a sedative on your first night because I'm going to wake you every 2 hours to check your blood pressure"
B. "You probably can't sleep at night because you take so many naps during the day"
C. "I'll call the physician to write an order for a sedative"
D. "A sedative might make your breathing too slow and shallow"

Answer sheet

A B C D	A B C D
1 ○ ○ ○ ○	31 ○ ○ ○ ○
2 ○ ○ ○ ○	32 ○ ○ ○ ○
3 ○ ○ ○ ○	33 ○ ○ ○ ○
4 ○ ○ ○ ○	34 ○ ○ ○ ○
5 ○ ○ ○ ○	35 ○ ○ ○ ○
6 ○ ○ ○ ○	36 ○ ○ ○ ○
7 ○ ○ ○ ○	37 ○ ○ ○ ○
8 ○ ○ ○ ○	38 ○ ○ ○ ○
9 ○ ○ ○ ○	39 ○ ○ ○ ○
10 ○ ○ ○ ○	40 ○ ○ ○ ○
11 ○ ○ ○ ○	41 ○ ○ ○ ○
12 ○ ○ ○ ○	42 ○ ○ ○ ○
13 ○ ○ ○ ○	43 ○ ○ ○ ○
14 ○ ○ ○ ○	44 ○ ○ ○ ○
15 ○ ○ ○ ○	45 ○ ○ ○ ○
16 ○ ○ ○ ○	46 ○ ○ ○ ○
17 ○ ○ ○ ○	47 ○ ○ ○ ○
18 ○ ○ ○ ○	48 ○ ○ ○ ○
19 ○ ○ ○ ○	49 ○ ○ ○ ○
20 ○ ○ ○ ○	50 ○ ○ ○ ○
21 ○ ○ ○ ○	51 ○ ○ ○ ○
22 ○ ○ ○ ○	52 ○ ○ ○ ○
23 ○ ○ ○ ○	53 ○ ○ ○ ○
24 ○ ○ ○ ○	54 ○ ○ ○ ○
25 ○ ○ ○ ○	55 ○ ○ ○ ○
26 ○ ○ ○ ○	
27 ○ ○ ○ ○	
28 ○ ○ ○ ○	
29 ○ ○ ○ ○	
30 ○ ○ ○ ○	

Answers and rationales

1 Correct answer—**C**

Pneumonia and atelectasis commonly cause capillary shunting, which occurs when pulmonary capillary blood comes in contact with totally unventilated alveoli; the shunt effect is perfusion in excess of ventilation. Mechanical deposits, such as dust or asbestos particles, are characteristic of such diseases as silicosis, a chronic disease that does not commonly lead to pneumonia or atelectasis. Anatomic dead space refers to the portion of the airway that is not involved in gas exchange (the nose and the trachea down to the bronchioles). Oxygen diffusion defect occurs when gas diffusion across the alveolar capillary membrane is altered by fluid surfactant or cellular trauma.

2 Correct answer—**A**

Several factors predispose an obese smoker undergoing upper abdominal surgery to pulmonary complications. An obese patient breathes shallowly; also, a high incision site exacerbates shallow breathing because of the pain caused by deep breaths. Smoking causes vasoconstriction and decreases ciliary action, impeding the removal of respiratory secretions. An upper abdominal surgery patient with normal pulmonary function has less risk of developing pulmonary complications than an obese smoker. A young lower abdominal surgery patient, even one with a chronic disease such as diabetes mellitus, also is less likely to have compromised pulmonary function. Unlike abdominal surgery, surgery on the extremities may not require general anesthesia, which commonly causes respiratory complications; also, a nonsmoking athlete probably has good pulmonary function, further lowering the risk of complications.

3 Correct answer—**C**

After upper abdominal surgery, a patient cannot take deep breaths or exhale forcefully because of splinting, postoperative pain, drainage tubes, and dressings. Therefore, vital capacity is decreased, and atelectasis and secretion accumulation may result. Because the patient cannot take deep breaths, tidal volume does not increase and lung compliance decreases. The patient's respiratory rate may change, but this usually is not significant.

4 Correct answer—**C**

An artificial airway—an endotracheal tube or, rarely, a tracheostomy tube—is established primarily to ventilate the patient and to remove secretions; this procedure also is performed to protect the airway of a comatose patient. Coughing can be stimulated without an artificial airway. Postural drainage is facilitated by proper positioning and bronchodilators, not by establishing an artificial airway. Vital capacity—the amount of air in a forced exhalation after maximum inhalation—cannot be changed with an artificial airway.

5 Correct answer—**C**

A patient with status asthmaticus occasionally develops acute respiratory failure late in an attack. This may occur with infections or pulmonary air leak, but it commonly occurs without evident complications. Exhaustion, coma, and deteriorating pulmonary function indicate lack of response to therapy or deterioration; altered arterial blood gas levels (partial pressure of carbon dioxide in arterial blood [$PaCO_2$] above 55 mm Hg, partial pressure of oxygen in arterial blood [PaO_2] below 50 mm Hg on 50% oxygen) indicate acute respiratory failure. The patient may require intubation and supportive ventilation. Acute pulmonary embolism causes initial sharp pain, hyperinflation, and respiratory alkalosis followed by respiratory acidosis. Acute pulmonary edema causes orthopnea, crackles, paroxysmal dyspnea, and pink, frothy sputum. Pneumonitis causes temperature elevation and purulent sputum.

6 Correct answer—**D**

Positive end-expiratory pressure (PEEP) is indicated when the patient's PaO_2 is less than 60 mm Hg with a fraction of inspired oxygen under 50%. PEEP maintains airway pressure greater than atmospheric pressure at the end of expiration; ventilator-applied PEEP exerts a constant, quantifiable force at the expiratory outlet of a breathing circuit. This increases functional residual capacity by increasing alveolar volumes or by reinflating previously collapsed alveoli. Increasing the respiratory rate or tidal volume might increase the PaO_2 but would also decrease the $PaCO_2$, putting the patient at risk for respiratory alkalosis. Increasing the driving pressure would increase the risk of alveolar rupture and subsequent pneumothorax.

7 Correct answer—**C**

A sputum smear and culture revealing tubercle bacilli under microscopic examination in the laboratory confirms tuberculosis (TB). Creatine kinase (CK) is one of the enzymes released into the serum by injured and damaged muscles; the presence of CK is not related to the diagnosis of TB. Chest X-ray can reveal changes in lung fields, such as tumors, inflammation, fractures, and fluid or air accumulation, but it does not confirm TB. The white blood cell (WBC) count increases with bacterial infection, but this does not confirm TB.

8 Correct answer—C

Productive cough, afternoon elevated temperature, hemoptysis, blood-streaked sputum, and night sweats are clinical manifestations of TB. Weight gain, dry cough, and urticaria have not been reported.

9 Correct answer—B

Speaking, coughing, or sneezing expels small droplets of moisture, which have small particles of respiratory secretions as nuclei. Some droplets fall to the ground; others are reduced by evaporation to dry particles that may stay in the air for long periods. Inhalation of air with the nuclei can cause infection of certain diseases, such as TB. Unlike other respiratory infections, however, TB does not require close contact (within 3 feet) or immediate exposure to the airborne nuclei for the disease to be transmitted; therefore, isolation techniques are necessary. People who have been exposed develop antibodies, but this does not necessarily mean they will not contract the disease.

10 Correct answer—B

By wearing a face mask that covers the nose and mouth, the nurse can prevent inhalation of tubercle bacilli. Rubber gloves and isolation gowns are indicated when direct contact with secretions containing the TB organism is possible, but like isolation booties, they have not demonstrated any effectiveness in preventing infection by airborne organisms; therefore, the nurse does not need to wear them at all times.

11 Correct answer—C

Range-of-motion exercises maintain joint mobility and muscle strength and prevent muscle atrophy in the patient on bed rest. Contact with family and friends is needed for the patient's psychological well-being, but because Mr. E. is on respiratory isolation, his contact should be restricted to close family during this highly infectious period. Mr. E. should not visit the lounge or other patients' rooms while on respiratory isolation.

12 Correct answer—C

Possible adverse effects of isoniazid (Laniazid) therapy include hepatic dysfunction, headache, vertigo, and peripheral neuritis. Tachycardia, insomnia, fever, GI dysfunction, and kidney damage have not been reported.

13 Correct answer—C

Drug therapy for TB lasts 9 to 12 months. The patient must understand that omission or irregular intake of isoniazid increases the possibility of microbial drug resistance, reversal of clinical improvement, and disease transmission to family members. Isoniazid does not cause nausea. The plan for Mr. E.'s regular follow-up care, the possible adverse effects of his medications, and the need to cover his nose and mouth with disposable tissues when coughing, sneezing, and laughing are important topics of discussion when providing discharge instructions.

14 Correct answer—B

Sarcoidosis, a systemic disease with multiple masses (granulomas) involving most organs, can affect the liver, spleen, heart, muscles, peripheral lymph nodes, mucous membranes, parotid glands, phalangeal bones, and nervous system. Some authorities believe sarcoidosis affects the immunologic system because T lymphocytes, which mediate immune activity in the lungs, occur in increased numbers. The disease is probably transmitted by an airborne antigen that causes an antibody reaction; it is not caused by air pollution associated with certain occupations. Although a high percentage of people with sarcoidosis are black, it is not a contagious disease nor a highly infectious disease of the respiratory tract.

15 Correct answer—A

Hypoglycemia is not an adverse effect of corticosteroids; possible effects include hyperglycemia, water retention, elevated blood pressure, changes in emotional states, and menstrual irregularities. The care plan should include orders to check blood glucose levels by fingerstick before meals and at bedtime to assess for hyperglycemia, to weigh the patient daily to assess for water retention, and to observe for mood swings.

16 Correct answer—D

Corticosteroids cause water retention and resultant weight gain in the body. Increasing salt intake will cause more water retention, leading to more weight gain and eventual complications, such as edema and hypertension. Oral prednisone (Deltasone), like any corticosteroid given for systemic effects, should not be discontinued abruptly because acute adrenal insufficiency may result. Corticosteroids may suppress the regenerative capacity of stomach mucosa, creating a potential increase in injury from stomach acid; taking the medication with food helps minimize this GI disturbance. Protection against infection is necessary because corticosteroids may reduce the body's resistance to infection.

17 Correct answer—B

Initial assessment of a patient with fractured ribs would reveal shallow breathing to minimize the pain accompanying any movement. Paradoxical respiration, in which the chest expands on expiration and contracts on inspiration, would be present only if the ribs sustained multiple fractures. Diminished breath sounds on the affected side would be present only if the patient had a pneumothorax. A clicking sensation during inspiration would be present only with costochondrial separation.

18 Correct answer—B

Hypoxia—insufficient oxygenation of the tissues—is characterized by restlessness, dyspnea, and tachycardia. Bradycardia, low blood pressure, and glycosuria are not signs of hypoxia.

19 Correct answer—A

Explaining that the tubes reinflate the collapsed portion of lung and make breathing easier should decrease the patient's fear of death. Assuring the patient that the nurse and physician will be present may reduce his anxiety, but not as much as a detailed explanation will. Notifying the physician to postpone the procedure is inappropriate because the chest tubes must be inserted immediately. Asking a priest to talk with the patient before the procedure may reduce the patient's anxiety and fears, but it would delay the procedure without increasing the patient's knowledge of the procedure.

20 Correct answer—C

Diazepam (Valium) relieves anxiety and tension related to organic or functional conditions. This drug has no analgesic effect. Because diazepam enhances muscle relaxation, it decreases muscle activity as well as respiratory rate.

21 Correct answer—A

A chest X-ray discloses the position of the tubes to determine the procedure's effectiveness. The X-ray is not done to advance the tube, although the physician may decide to adjust the tube after reviewing the X-ray. Tomography—used to study cavities, neoplasms, and lung densities—visualizes a single layer of the lungs. An ultrasound or echogram records sound waves that penetrate the lungs.

22 Correct answer—A

Bubbling in the water-seal chamber may indicate an air leak in the system, which predisposes the patient to tension pneumothorax. Fluctuation of fluid in the water-seal chamber is normal unless the lung has reexpanded, suctioning is not working, or tubes are obstructed. Dark red drainage, indicating previous bleeding caused by trauma, is expected; bright red drainage, indicating fresh bleeding, should be reported immediately. The drainage device was set at 20 cm of suction, so a fluid level of 20 cm in the suction control chamber is normal.

23 Correct answer—C

Positioning the patient on his right side is inappropriate because his fractured ribs are on this side; this position would increase the patient's pain, interfering with chest expansion. Coughing, deep breathing, and using an incentive spirometer help inflate the lungs and remove secretions, thereby improving pulmonary ventilation. Hydration makes secretions less viscous and tenacious, which enhances their removal and improves ventilation.

24 Correct answer—D

A chest X-ray must confirm lung reexpansion before chest tubes can be removed. The amount of chest tube drainage and the cessation of pain and dyspnea are not indications for removal. The presence of the chest tubes themselves may be irritating and painful; the pain may increase the patient's dyspnea. Absence of fluid fluctuation in the water-seal chamber may indicate that the lung has reexpanded, but it also could mean that the chest tubes are obstructed or the drainage device is not working.

25 Correct answer—D

Valsalva's maneuver causes a bearing-down effect, increasing pressure throughout the body and preventing air from entering the pleural cavity. Breathing through pursed lips, quickly and shallowly, or with an open mouth will not prevent air from entering when chest tubes are removed.

26 Correct answer—A

After a bronchoscopy, the gag reflex must be present to prevent aspiration of food or fluid into the lungs. Abdominal distention, dyspnea, and dyspepsia are not related to the presence of the gag reflex.

27 Correct answer—D

Pulmonary function tests, which measure lung volume and capacity, help identify the degree of respiratory disability. The results indicate whether enough functioning lung tissue will be intact after surgery to compensate for the removal of diseased tissue. Pulmonary function tests are not used to evaluate the spread of the disease, estimate the amount of anesthesia needed for surgery, or determine how much tissue needs to be removed.

28 Correct answer—D

A normal respiratory rate (less than 20 breaths/minute) without dyspnea indicates probable lung expansion and effective chest tube functioning. Reporting less chest pain or requesting more pain medication would be more appropriate patient outcomes for a nursing diagnosis of *Pain related to lung impairment and chest surgery.* Assuming a semi-Fowler's position, which facilitates breathing, may indicate that gas exchange is still impaired.

29 Correct answer—B

If the patient washes off the marks placed on the skin to guide radiation therapy, the areas must be reassessed and remarked—a time-consuming task. Skin lotions and powders are contraindicated because they may irritate the skin in the irradiated area. The patient should avoid wearing constrictive clothing, which decreases circulation. Massaging an area already tender from radiation can cause irritation and pain.

30 Correct answer—C

Because Mr. B.'s loss of appetite causes him to eat less than normal, he should make every mouthful count by eating high-calorie foods. Moderate activity increases a person's appetite. Forcing fluids typically causes a feeling of fullness; this would further reduce the patient's appetite and nutritional intake. He should avoid hot meat dishes, which commonly cause a metallic taste in the patient receiving radiation therapy.

31 Correct answer—D

Chronic obstructive pulmonary disease (COPD) can cause hypoxemia and pulmonary hypertension. Hypoxemia causes increased production of red blood cells, making the blood more viscous. The increased viscosity combined with increased pulmonary pressure forces the right side of the heart to work harder than usual, result-

ing in right ventricular hypertrophy. Ankle edema is a common assessment finding of this condition. The right atrium may decompen-
sate as the hypertrophy worsens; the left atrium and left ventricle
are not affected.

32 Correct answer—C

A high carbon dioxide (CO_2) level is the normal stimulus for
breathing. A patient with COPD chronically retains CO_2. When this
retention occurs over a long period, high levels of CO_2 will no
longer stimulate the brain's respiratory centers; they then become
stimulated by a low partial pressure of oxygen in arterial blood
(PaO_2). If oxygen is administered at levels greater than 2 liters/min-
ute, the patient's PaO_2 increases and eliminates the stimulus to
breathe. The other statements concerning oxygen therapy are true
but do not relate specifically to oxygen therapy and COPD.

33 Correct answer—B

Aminophylline (Aminophyllin), a bronchodilator, belongs to the xanthine category of drugs. Toxic reactions to xanthines include tachycardia, nausea and vomiting, insomnia, anxiety, and nervousness.
Depression, lethargy, and cyanosis are not symptoms of xanthine
toxicity.

34 Correct answer—B

The pH, which is less than 7.35, reflects acidosis; the $PaCO_2$ value is
above normal (35 to 45 mm Hg), indicating that the imbalance origi-
nates in the respiratory system. The normal HCO_3^- level means that
renal compensation, always slow in onset, has not yet begun. Respiratory acidosis is caused by CO_2 retention; it occurs commonly in patients with obstructive lung disease.

35 Correct answer—C

For a patient with COPD, a hot drink in the morning typically helps
to liquefy pulmonary secretions that have pooled overnight so that
they can be expectorated. Congestion and variable wheezing are expected in a patient with COPD; taking vital signs, calling the physician, or checking heart sounds would be inappropriate.

36 Correct answer—A

During pursed-lip breathing, the patient takes twice as long to exhale. This empties the lungs of CO_2 more completely and helps the
patient control respirations when anxious or during respiratory distress. Coughing technique, postural drainage, and relaxation tech-

niques are important matters to teach any patient with a respiratory disorder, but pursed-lip breathing would best alleviate Mr. J.'s inability to exhale efficiently.

37 Correct answer—A

In postural drainage, the patient's positioning allows gravity to help drain specific lung segments of retained secretions, which are coughed up or removed by suctioning. The patient's positioning differs according to which lung segments need draining. Rhythmic clapping of the chest wall with cupped hands is called percussion. Postural drainage, which is performed before meals, should be performed only as long as the patient can tolerate it.

38 Correct answer—D

Cyanosis is a late sign of increased or retained CO_2 and decreased oxygen, indicating impaired gas exchange. Mrs. Z.'s altered comfort may lead to reduced chest movement and shallow breathing, further decreasing CO_2 expiration and O_2 intake; however, this is not the cause of the cyanosis. The information is insufficient to consider anemia or cardiac problems as the cause.

39 Correct answer—A

With decreased oxygen to the brain, cells shift to anaerobic metabolism, which produces lactic acid and cell death. This affects the central nervous system (CNS), causing irritability. Cerebral hypoxia also causes drowsiness, not hyperactivity or mental alertness. Frequent urination may indicate an unrelated problem.

40 Correct answer—B

The rectal route typically provides an accurate temperature reading because of the rectum's large blood supply and the relative ease in maintaining contact between the thermometer and the mucosa. The oral route may not provide an accurate reading because the patient is coughing and breathing through the mouth, interfering with contact between the thermometer and mucosa. The axillary route is the least accurate method, especially for a patient with a severe respiratory infection, and accurate temperature readings are essential for this patient.

41 Correct answer—B

Codeine is used in antitussive medications to decrease the frequency and intensity of coughing without eliminating the protective cough reflex. Codeine does not suppress the gag reflex. When coughing is lessened, tracheal irritation decreases, but this is a secondary drug effect. Codeine does decrease chest pain, but this is not its primary purpose in an antitussive medication.

42 Correct answer—B

Water vapor makes respiratory secretions less thick and tenacious so they are easier for the patient to cough up. Postural drainage will not loosen the secretions if they are extremely thick. Coughing and deep breathing every hour will help move the secretions, but only after they have been loosened. Milk may increase the tenaciousness of respiratory secretions.

43 Correct answer—B

Sputum, the exudate produced by inflammation and infection in the lungs, is examined because it may contain microorganisms causing the tissue response. Spitting saliva and surface mucus into the container would contaminate the sputum specimen. Nasal secretions, which may be present in the nose and throat, normally harbor their own microorganisms; clearing the nose and throat helps prevent contamination of the sputum specimen. The patient should deep-breathe to expand and aerate the lung tissue and then use diaphragmatic contractions to propel respiratory secretions upward into the trachea or mouth.

44 Correct answer—C

Because respiratory secretions pool and accumulate from inactivity while the patient sleeps, a sputum specimen obtained in the morning will contain less saliva. If the specimen is obtained at other times of the day, its volume and consistency may vary with the treatments received. Unless sputum is loose and copious, treatment may be needed to liquefy or loosen secretions to obtain a specimen.

45 Correct answer—C

Rust-colored sputum indicates bacterial pneumonia. Bright red sputum indicates active bleeding in the lung tissue; pink-tinged sputum suggests a lung tumor. Thin, mucoid sputum may indicate viral pneumonia.

46 Correct answer—A

Streptococcus pneumoniae is the most common cause of bacterial pneumonia. It is most prevalent during the winter and spring. *Proteus* bacteria are found in fecal material. *Haemophilus influenzae* causes viral pneumonia. *Escherichia coli* is normally found in the intestinal tract.

47 Correct answer—C

Many vaccines, such as the influenza vaccine, are made with egg or chick embryo; therefore, a person allergic to eggs may have dangerous reactions to these vaccines. The influenza vaccination will not endanger a person sensitive to the other allergens listed.

48 Correct answer—B

When pneumothorax is present during airway pressure therapy, a chest tube must be inserted to drain accumulated fluid from the pleural cavity. A perfusion scan evaluates the patient's respiratory function but does not resolve the pneumothorax, which is the immediate priority. Positive end-expiratory pressure therapy may worsen the patient's condition; maintaining high end-expiratory airway pressures could lead to rupture of the bullae. An electrocardiogram provides information related to the heart's electrical activity; the data provided do not indicate any cardiac irregularities.

49 Correct answer—D

Septicemia is not associated with these nursing actions; the other three responses are possible complications. Most patients in acute respiratory failure are ventilated with supplemental oxygen to achieve an acceptable PaO_2. When a catheter is placed in the airway and a vacuum applied, oxygen-enriched air is sucked out and replaced by room air, resulting in moderate to severe hypoxemia. This hypoxemia can cause cardiac arrhythmias and even cardiac arrest; hypotension and lung collapse also may occur. Suctioning should be performed after giving the patient oxygen and then only intermittently for a short period, using appropriate medical asepsis.

50 Correct answer—A

The peak inspiratory pressure is measured by attaching an aneroid manometer to the endotracheal or tracheostomy tube and then having the patient, after a maximal exhalation, inhale as forcefully as possible. Negative pressure greater than -20 cm H_2O indicates adequate inspiratory muscle strength. The vital capacity can be measured easily with a respirometer. The vital capacity should be greater than 10 ml/kg of body weight to avoid atelectasis. Arterial oxygenation (PaO_2) on 100% oxygen would be close to 600 mm Hg in a person with normal respiratory functioning. An increase in shunt fraction indicates a worsening condition, which would preclude weaning.

51 Correct answer—D

Anxiety is not a critical factor requiring improvement before weaning the patient from the ventilator. Factors that must be improved before weaning include acid-base abnormalities, anemias, caloric depletion, fever, fluid imbalance, infection, hyperglycemia, reduced cardiac output, renal failure, and a decreased level of consciousness.

52 Correct answer—A

Obesity hypoventilation syndrome (OHS) causes alveolar hypoventilation with marked depression of the normal ventilatory response to increasing serum CO_2 levels. This increase in CO_2 stimulates the medulla, causing the respirations to become shallow and rapid. Aminophylline acts directly on the bronchial smooth muscles, causing bronchodilation. This allows more air to enter the lungs and stimulates the CNS, increasing the breathing reflex. Aminophylline does not affect respiratory rate, depth, or secretions.

53 Correct answer—C

Toxic doses of aminophylline stimulate the CNS and may cause headache, tachycardia, palpitations, hypertension, arrhythmias, nervousness, irritability, restlessness, muscle twitching, and nausea.

54 Correct answer—A

Assessment of rate, depth, and pattern of breathing is the nurse's top priority when caring for a patient with OHS; the nurse's short-term goal is to correct the respiratory acidosis produced by alveolar hypoventilation. The patient with OHS may have an upper airway obstruction from fatty deposits of the pharynx or from a short, thick neck; also, obesity increases the work of breathing and may impair thoracic movements. Nutritional intake is considered only after the acute respiratory problem is stabilized. OHS does not cause life-threatening cardiovascular or neurovascular problems, so these assessments are not a priority.

55 Correct answer—D

The physician specifically ordered no sedatives for this patient because of the risk of respiratory failure. OHS makes the patient's breathing slower and shallower. This causes an increase in CO_2 retention and hypoxemia, leading to central apnea. Sedatives are contraindicated in the obese patient with central apnea because they may precipitate respiratory failure. The other responses are inappropriate.

CHAPTER 2

Cardiovascular System

Questions

1 Which measure is most important for a patient with thromboangiitis obliterans (Buerger's disease)?

A. Protecting the extremities from trauma
B. Maintaining adequate hydration
C. Quitting smoking
D. Protecting the extremities from chilling and exposure

2 Which statement does *not* accurately describe thromboangiitis obliterans?

A. It is an occlusive disease of small- and medium-sized arteries
B. It typically affects young male cigarette smokers
C. Its possible complications include ulceration and gangrene
D. Its first symptom usually is chest pain

3 Intermittent claudication refers to:

A. Leg pain that occurs after exercise and is relieved after rest
B. Nonhealing ulcers on the lower leg near the ankle
C. Pain in the calf or foot that occurs at rest
D. Burning or cold sensation that increases with exercise and is relieved by elevating the legs

4 Intermittent claudication is an indication of which condition?

A. Phlebitis
B. Arterial insufficiency
C. Venous insufficiency
D. Mitral regurgitation

5 While reading a patient's chart, the nurse sees pedal pulses described as 4+ bilaterally. This indicates that the pulses are:

A. Thready and weak
B. Slightly impaired
C. Unequal
D. Normal

6 While auscultating a patient's femoral area, the nurse notes a bruit. Bruits are caused by:

A. Turbulent blood flow through stenotic blood vessels
B. Occluded blood vessels
C. Hypotension when the patient arises
D. Development of collateral circulation

7 A patient is scheduled for an impedance plethysmography study. This procedure identifies:

A. Obstruction of arterial inflow
B. Obstruction of venous outflow
C. Distal aneurysms
D. Arteriosclerosis obliterans

8 While caring for a patient who recently had surgery, the nurse realizes that he is at risk for venous thrombosis. Which measure would help prevent venous thrombosis?

A. Avoiding ambulation
B. Hyperflexing the knees
C. Moving and exercising the leg frequently
D. Avoiding the use of support stockings

9 Mr. M., a 65-year-old diabetic patient with arterial insufficiency in the legs, complains that his feet are cold. Which nursing measure is contraindicated?

A. Applying a heating pad to the patient's feet
B. Applying warm socks
C. Encouraging exercise
D. Increasing the room temperature slightly

10 Which statement does *not* accurately describe Raynaud's disease?

A. It is characterized by episodic digital vasospasm associated with skin color changes
B. It is precipitated by exposure to cold or by emotional stress
C. It typically is seen in the fingers and toes
D. It usually occurs in men ages 40 to 60

11 Which finding would the nurse expect when examining a patient with a diagnosis of abdominal aortic aneurysm?

A. Tachycardia
B. Pulsatile abdominal mass
C. Paresis of the legs
D. Carotid bruits

12 A patient is scheduled for surgical repair of an abdominal aortic aneurysm. Which preoperative complication presents the greatest threat to the patient?

A. Embolism in the foot
B. Rupture of the aneurysm
C. Cerebrovascular accident
D. Myocardial infarction

SITUATION

Mr. A., age 68, is admitted with a diagnosis of arteriosclerosis obliterans.

Questions 13 to 16 refer to this situation.

13 While assessing Mr. A., the nurse is unable to palpate a pulse on the top of his foot. She would report that she cannot palpate the:

A. Popliteal pulse
B. Posterior tibial pulse
C. Femoral pulse
D. Dorsalis pedis pulse

14 Which symptom indicates the most severe ischemia in a patient with arteriosclerosis obliterans?

A. Rest pain
B. Trophic changes
C. Gangrene of the toes
D. Disabling claudication

15 The nurse preparing a teaching plan for Mr. A. should base her instructions on which description of arteriosclerosis obliterans?

A. It is a rapidly progressing disease with no symptoms in its early stages
B. It is a chronic, slowly developing disease that becomes symptomatic after blood flow is significantly reduced
C. It is not considered a systemic disease and most often affects only a small area of the body
D. The most severe symptoms usually occur during the disease's early stages

16 Which statement by Mr. A. would indicate a need for further instructions?

A. "I have quit smoking"
B. "I make sure to dry my feet thoroughly"
C. "I haven't taken a walk for weeks"
D. "I am trying to lose weight because I'm too heavy"

SITUATION

Mrs. G., age 35, is admitted with a diagnosis of thrombophlebitis of the left leg.

Questions 17 to 21 refer to this situation.

17 The nurse takes leg measurements to detect swelling. All of the following actions are appropriate *except:*

A. Taking measurements with the patient in a dorsal recumbent position
B. Using a felt-tipped pen to mark the position of the measuring tape on the patient's legs
C. Taking measurements with the patient standing
D. Taking bilateral measurements

18 The most likely manifestation of thrombophlebitis in Mrs. G. is:

A. Calf pain
B. Foot drop
C. Bilateral ankle edema
D. Varicose veins

19 Which nursing measure is contraindicated while caring for Mrs. G.?

A. Maintaining bed rest
B. Massaging the affected leg
C. Elevating the legs on pillows
D. Encouraging fluid intake

20 Which finding should the nurse report immediately when assessing Mrs. G.?

A. Shortness of breath
B. Increased skin temperature of the affected leg
C. Calf tenderness
D. Reddened skin

21 When instructing Mrs. G. on the proper use of support stockings, the nurse should tell her to:

A. Apply them in the evening before sleeping
B. Roll down the top of the stockings to the desired length
C. Apply them in the morning before ambulation
D. Remove them only once a week

SITUATION

Mr. T., age 63, is admitted to the hospital with a diagnosis of congestive heart failure (CHF). The physician's orders include 500 mg of chlorothiazide (Diuril) P.O. twice daily and 0.25 mg of digoxin (Lanoxin) P.O. daily.

Questions 22 to 26 refer to this situation.

22 Assessment of Mr. T. would most likely reveal:

A. Crushing chest pain unrelieved by rest or nitroglycerin (Nitro-Bid)
B. Diaphoresis with cool, clammy skin
C. Distended neck veins and dependent pitting edema
D. Fever and an elevated white blood cell count

23 Mr. T. is in the acute phase of ventricular heart failure. To alleviate his symptoms, the nurse should place him in:

A. The dorsal recumbent position with elevated feet to reduce edema
B. An upright position to promote chest expansion
C. The low-Fowler's position with elevated knees to slow the return of blood to the heart
D. The left lateral Sims' position to promote emptying to the right side of the heart

24 The nurse administers chlorothiazide. This drug should alleviate Mr. T.'s symptoms by:

A. Reducing circulatory volume through diuresis
B. Strengthening the force of ventricular contractions
C. Reducing the rate of metabolism and the body's need for oxygen
D. Slowing the rate of heart contractions

25 Mr. T. is placed on a strict low-sodium, high-potassium diet. Which lunch menu is most appropriate for him?

A. Bologna sandwich on low-sodium bread, carrot sticks, orange, and skim milk
B. Tuna fish, noodle and vegetable casserole, banana, and coffee
C. Boiled egg sandwich on low-sodium toast; lettuce, tomato, and onion salad; banana; and skim milk
D. Chicken sandwich on low-sodium bread, celery sticks, apple, and tea with lemon

26 When assessing Mr. T. for signs and symptoms of digoxin toxicity, the nurse should watch for all of the following *except:*

A. Bradycardia, tachycardia, bigeminy, ectopic beats, and pulse deficits
B. Anorexia, nausea and vomiting, diarrhea, and abdominal pain
C. Headache, double or blurred vision, drowsiness, confusion, restlessness, and muscle weakness
D. Abdominal distention, weakness, paralysis, apathy, depression, and hallucinations

SITUATION

Mr. S., a 66-year-old patient with stable essential hypertension, is admitted to the hospital after returning home from vacation. He states he lost his blood pressure medications the first day of his vacation and didn't replace them. On admission, his blood pressure is 200/130 mm Hg.

Questions 27 to 29 refer to this situation.

27 Which results should the nurse expect on review of Mr. S.'s admission laboratory studies?

A. Protein and red blood cells (RBCs) in the urine
B. Lowered blood urea nitrogen and creatinine levels
C. Elevated blood glucose level
D. Normal size and shape of RBCs

28 During afternoon rounds, the nurse notices Mr. S. has a decreased level of consciousness. He complains of a persistent headache that has been increasing in severity. Examination reveals unequal pupils, strong peripheral pulses, and a blood pressure of 180/120 mm Hg. The nurse should suspect that:

A. The patient is experiencing adverse effects from his antihypertensive medication
B. He has hypertensive encephalopathy caused by cerebral ischemia and edema
C. Excessive arterial vascular pressure has caused a thromboembolism
D. Excessive intravascular pressure has caused an aneurysm to rupture

29 All of the following measures would increase Mr. S.'s compliance with treatment *except:*

A. Helping him identify ways to incorporate treatments into his present life-style
B. Encouraging him to participate in a support group for hypertensive individuals
C. Supporting his decision to continue smoking if it relaxes him
D. Providing written instructions

SITUATION

Mrs. J., a 58-year-old patient with long-standing hypertension, is admitted for shortness of breath. During morning rounds, the nurse notices that Mrs. J. has developed an S_4 gallop, crackles, and diminished breath sounds, which indicate CHF.

Questions 30 to 33 refer to this situation.

30 The nursing care plan for Mrs. J. should include:

A. Positioning the patient flat in bed
B. Elevating the head of the bed and providing a calm, restful environment
C. Elevating the knees to promote venous flow
D. Encouraging the patient to perform Valsalva's maneuver when necessary

31 Mrs. J.'s orders include a low-sodium diet and drug therapy with furosemide (Lasix), hydralazine (Apresoline), and digoxin (Lanoxin). After administering furosemide to Mrs. J. and before administering digoxin, the nurse should review laboratory test results for:

A. High sodium levels
B. Low uric acid levels
C. High blood lipid levels
D. Low potassium levels

32 Which statement indicates that Mrs. J. understands her discharge instructions?

A. "I will avoid tomatoes, oranges, and bananas; these will interfere with my diuretic therapy"
B. "I should avoid aerobic exercise, but weight lifting is OK"
C. "Hypertension is a lifelong problem; I will need to take my medication every day from now on"
D. "Canned and frozen vegetables and soups are the best to buy for my diet"

33 Mrs. J. is admitted a year later with a diagnosis of malignant hypertension. Which drugs commonly are used to treat this disorder?

A. Beta blockers and angiotensin converting enzyme (ACE) inhibitors administered orally
B. ACE inhibitors and diuretics administered orally
C. Adrenergic blockers and vasodilators administered intravenously
D. Vasodilators and diuretics administered intravenously

SITUATION

Ms. L., a 26-year-old patient with a history of mitral valve stenosis, is admitted to a medical unit complaining of anorexia, fatigue, and a low-grade fever of 100.2° to 100.4° F (37.9° to 38° C) that has lasted for a week. She states she had a root canal done 1 month ago. A blood culture and an echocardiogram confirm a diagnosis of subacute bacterial endocarditis (SBE).

Questions 34 to 37 refer to this situation.

34 Which statement best describes the pathophysiology of mitral valve stenosis?

A. The mitral valve atrophies, leading to atrial dilation and hypertrophy
B. A fibrous ring forms around the mitral valve, causing backflow of blood into the atrium
C. Chordae tendineae become shorter and thicker, and valve leaflets fuse
D. The mitral valve leaflets widen, and the flaps are unable to close completely

35 Physical assessment of Ms. L. might reveal all of the following findings *except:*

A. A loud S_1 heart sound
B. Adventitious lung sounds
C. A loud S_2 heart sound
D. Peripheral edema

36 All of the following signs and symptoms indicate a complication of SBE *except:*

A. Intractable vomiting
B. Left upper quadrant pain
C. Hematuria
D. Hypotension

37 When preparing Ms. L. for discharge, the nurse should discuss all of the following topics *except:*

A. Maintaining bed rest for 2 to 4 weeks
B. Continuing to take prescribed antibiotics for 4 to 6 weeks
C. Requesting prophylactic antibiotics before dental or gynecologic procedures
D. Recognizing signs and symptoms of possible relapse

SITUATION

Mr. J., a 44-year-old banker, comes to the hospital with complaints of mild chest pain that radiates to his left arm and jaw. He was mowing his lawn when the pain began, and it subsided after he sat down. He states that he had a similar episode several days earlier after eating dinner, which he thought was caused by indigestion.

Questions 38 to 48 refer to this situation.

38 The nurse assesses Mr. J. for coronary risk factors. Which finding obtained during the health history represents the greatest risk?

A. The patient's brother had a myocardial infarction (MI), and his sister has hypertension
B. The patient has smoked one pack of cigarettes per day for 20 years
C. The patient has a sedentary life-style
D. The patient works long hours in a stressful environment

39 Mr. J. is scheduled for a resting thallium myocardial scan. During preprocedural teaching, the nurse should tell Mr. J. that this scan:

A. Is noninvasive
B. Detects areas of perfusion in the myocardium
C. Determines coronary artery insufficiency during exercise
D. Eliminates the need for cardiac catheterization

40 The physician diagnoses angina pectoris. The nurse instructs Mr. J. in the differences between angina and MI pain. Which statement is *not* true of angina?

A. It indicates periods of coronary insufficiency
B. It is localized in the chest and left arm
C. It usually lasts less than 10 minutes
D. It is relieved with rest or nitroglycerin

41 When Mr. J. is discharged, his drug regimen is 30 mg of diltiazem (Cardizem) P.O. three times daily, 20 mg of isosorbide dinitrate (Isordil) P.O. four times daily, and 0.15 mg of nitroglycerin (Nitro-Bid) sublingually as needed. The nurse informs Mr. J. of the actions, adverse effects, and correct storage and use of these medications. Which statement shows that Mr. J. understands this information?

A. "All three of these drugs will help improve blood flow to my heart"
B. "I can keep my daily doses in this plastic pill box"
C. "I shouldn't have any more pain with these pills"
D. "The nitroglycerin will lower my blood pressure"

42 Six months after discharge, Mr. J. is admitted to the emergency department (ED) with severe chest and arm pain of 4 hours' duration, accompanied by sweating and weakness. While assessing Mr. J, the nurse should first try to relieve his discomfort by:

A. Administering 4 mg of morphine I.V.
B. Checking his arterial blood gas levels
C. Instructing him in guided imagery
D. Starting oxygen by nasal cannula at 2 liters/minute

43 The ED nurse takes an electrocardiogram (ECG), which shows sinus tachycardia (124 heart beats/minute); marked ST-segment elevation in leads I, II, and V_1 through V_5; slight T-wave inversion in leads I and V_1 through V_3; Q waves of 2 to 4 mm in V_1 through V_3; and 6 to 7 premature ventricular contractions (PVCs) per minute. The physician diagnoses an acute anterior MI. Which waveform pattern indicates a currently evolving MI?

A. PVCs
B. Q waves
C. ST-segment depression
D. ST-segment elevation and T-wave inversion

44 When Mr. J. arrives in the coronary care unit (CCU), the nurse reviews his ECGs and laboratory test results. Which result most accurately confirms that the patient has suffered an MI?

A. Elevated MB isoenzyme of creatine phosphokinase (CPK-MB) level
B. Elevated lactate dehydrogenase level
C. Elevated erythrocyte sedimentation rate
D. Elevated serum aspartate aminotransferase (formerly glutamic-oxaloacetic transaminase) level

45 Mr. J.'s heart rate is 96 beats/minute, and he is still having frequent PVCs. His physician orders a bolus of 100 mg of lidocaine (Xylocaine), followed by a 2 mg/minute drip of 2 g of lidocaine in 500 ml of dextrose 5% in water to be titrated p.r.n. to 4 mg/minute. His ECG begins to show malignant (or significant) PVCs, in which:

A. P waves follow the PVCs
B. The PVCs are farther apart, with 10 normal QRS complexes between each one
C. The PVCs fall on or near the T wave
D. The PVCs fall on the P wave

46 Mr. J.'s pain is relieved 4 hours after admission. He states that he feels much better and "should probably go home tomorrow—these angina attacks aren't really serious." Which stage of grief does this statement indicate Mr. J. is experiencing?

A. Acceptance
B. Bargaining
C. Denial
D. Depression

47 After 3 days in the CCU with no further complications, Mr. J. is sent to the coronary step-down unit. He is scheduled for a left-sided retrograde cardiac catheterization on the tenth day after his MI. Preparations for the procedure would include:

A. Administering heparin
B. Explaining what occurs during femoral vein cannulation
C. Maintaining the patient on nothing-by-mouth status for 24 hours before the procedure
D. Questioning the patient about allergies

48 During the cardiac catheterization, Mr. J.'s MI extends to the inferior portion of his myocardium, and he exhibits signs and symptoms of cardiogenic shock. All of the following are characteristic of cardiogenic shock *except:*

A. Disorientation to time and place
B. Narrowed pulse pressure and thready pulse
C. Pain in the distal, left lower extremity
D. ECG showing ST-segment elevations in leads II, III, and aV_F

SITUATION

Mrs. S., a 76-year-old retired school teacher, arrives at the ED accompanied by her daughter. She complains she has been experiencing "sinking spells." When asked for clarification, her daughter states that Mrs. S. occasionally blacks out briefly during conversations and that she found her mother unconscious on the bathroom floor that morning.

Questions 49 to 52 refer to this situation.

49 The nurse connects Mrs. S. to the cardiac monitor. Initially, her ECG strip shows a PR interval of 0.26 second; atrial and ventricular rates of 54 beats/minute; and one to three unifocal PVCs/minute, with compensatory pauses following each one. These findings indicate:

A. Bradycardia with first-degree atrioventricular (AV) block
B. Bradycardia with second-degree AV block
C. Complete heart block with ventricular escape beats
D. Normal sinus rhythm with occasional PVCs

50 The physician places Mrs. S. on a Holter monitor on the medical unit and allows her to continue most of her normal activities. The nurse explains to her that the monitoring:

A. Correlates activities and heart response by using a diary and taped ECG
B. Denotes an ischemic response while on the treadmill
C. Indicates valvular outlines on the monitor and correlates them with heart sounds
D. Highlights "cold" spots on the imaging screen

51 After analyzing Mrs. S.'s Holter monitor results, the physician diagnoses sick sinus syndrome with Stokes-Adams attacks and decides to insert a permanent ventricular pacemaker the next morning. The evening nurse explains to Mrs. S. the changes she must make in her activities after receiving her pacemaker, including:

A. No heavy lifting for 6 months
B. Brisk exercise to improve collateral circulation
C. Curtailment of her needlework and daily walk
D. Some limitations of vigorous upper extremity movements

52 The nurse reviews discharge instructions with Mrs. S. Which statement indicates that Mrs. S. may not completely understand her instructions?

A. "I'll take my pulse every morning and write it on this chart"
B. "If I have a little bit of clear drainage from my wound for a few weeks, I shouldn't be alarmed about it"
C. "I've ordered a medical alert bracelet with my pacemaker information on it"
D. "My daughter is buying me a new microwave oven—mine is one of those older models that might not be safe"

SITUATION

Mr. P., a 57-year-old steelworker with a history of angina, has been having more frequent attacks of chest pain. He is admitted to the ED with chest pain unrelieved by three nitroglycerin tablets. The physician diagnoses Prinzmetal's variant angina.

Questions 53 to 58 refer to this situation.

53 The diagnosis of Prinzmetal's variant angina means that the patient's pain:

A. Is unresponsive to most therapies
B. Occurs most frequently during rest
C. Occurs in paroxysms while reclining
D. Occurs most frequently during REM sleep

54 Mr. P. is discharged home with instructions to report to the medical clinic the following day for a cardiac catheterization. After this procedure, the physician diagnoses three-vessel disease with inoperable distal lesions. Which statement by Mr. P. best demonstrates to the nurse that he understands his diagnosis?

A. "I'd better update my will; I don't have long to live"
B. "I'll have to quit my job and take an early retirement pension"
C. "My brother said there's a doctor in Denver who can cure the kind of disease that I have"
D. "With medication, diet, and mild exercise, I should last a few more years"

55 Mr. P. asks his primary nurse whether he and his wife should continue to have sex. The nurse's most appropriate response would be:

A. "Your wife may be hesitant because she's afraid of causing you pain"
B. "The frustration of abstaining is more likely to cause chest pain than intercourse is"
C. "Maybe you should discuss it with your physician"
D. "You may try a different position or time of day if you begin to have chest pain"

56 Two years later, Mr. P. is readmitted with a subendocardial MI. Which statement about subendocardial MI is correct?

A. It involves a small portion of the inferior outer layer of the heart muscle and may cause irritation of the diaphragm
B. Although considered relatively mild, it involves the entire outer layer of the myocardium
C. Although considered relatively mild, it may extend and involve larger areas of the myocardium
D. It is a very severe MI that involves large areas of the myocardium and carries a poor prognosis

57 Mr. P.'s MI extends, and he begins to show signs of left ventricular failure. Which sign would appear first?

A. An S_4 heart sound
B. Crackles and cough
C. An S_3 heart sound
D. Pink, frothy sputum

58 The left ventricular failure worsens, and Mr. P.'s physician orders dopamine (Intropin) and nitroprusside I.V. drips. The CCU nurse who transcribes these orders should:

A. Call the physician and tell him that these two drugs are incompatible
B. Titrate the two drugs to maintain the patient's blood pressure within an ordered range
C. Obtain an order for additional morphine, because these two drugs cause severe localized pain
D. Plan to administer the drugs via a single I.V. site in the hand

Answer sheet

	A B C D		A B C D
1	○ ○ ○ ○	31	○ ○ ○ ○
2	○ ○ ○ ○	32	○ ○ ○ ○
3	○ ○ ○ ○	33	○ ○ ○ ○
4	○ ○ ○ ○	34	○ ○ ○ ○
5	○ ○ ○ ○	35	○ ○ ○ ○
6	○ ○ ○ ○	36	○ ○ ○ ○
7	○ ○ ○ ○	37	○ ○ ○ ○
8	○ ○ ○ ○	38	○ ○ ○ ○
9	○ ○ ○ ○	39	○ ○ ○ ○
10	○ ○ ○ ○	40	○ ○ ○ ○
11	○ ○ ○ ○	41	○ ○ ○ ○
12	○ ○ ○ ○	42	○ ○ ○ ○
13	○ ○ ○ ○	43	○ ○ ○ ○
14	○ ○ ○ ○	44	○ ○ ○ ○
15	○ ○ ○ ○	45	○ ○ ○ ○
16	○ ○ ○ ○	46	○ ○ ○ ○
17	○ ○ ○ ○	47	○ ○ ○ ○
18	○ ○ ○ ○	48	○ ○ ○ ○
19	○ ○ ○ ○	49	○ ○ ○ ○
20	○ ○ ○ ○	50	○ ○ ○ ○
21	○ ○ ○ ○	51	○ ○ ○ ○
22	○ ○ ○ ○	52	○ ○ ○ ○
23	○ ○ ○ ○	53	○ ○ ○ ○
24	○ ○ ○ ○	54	○ ○ ○ ○
25	○ ○ ○ ○	55	○ ○ ○ ○
26	○ ○ ○ ○	56	○ ○ ○ ○
27	○ ○ ○ ○	57	○ ○ ○ ○
28	○ ○ ○ ○	58	○ ○ ○ ○
29	○ ○ ○ ○		
30	○ ○ ○ ○		

Answers and rationales

1 Correct answer—**C**

Nicotine in tobacco causes vasoconstriction; if the patient continues to smoke, the disease progresses. The other measures listed are appropriate for the patient with thromboangiitis obliterans but are not as important as avoiding tobacco. Maintaining adequate hydration helps prevent hemoconcentration and clot formation. Protecting the extremities from trauma is necessary because impaired circulation causes poor healing. Because the disease causes some neuropathy that decreases sensitivity to temperature changes, the extremities must be protected from chilling and exposure to prevent injuries the patient may not sense.

2 Correct answer—**D**

Chest pain is not the first symptom of thromboangiitis obliterans, although it may occur as the disease progresses if the coronary arteries are affected. Thromboangiitis obliterans is an occlusive disease of small- and medium-sized arteries that eventually affects the veins as well. It typically causes intermittent claudication of the instep, which is aggravated by exercise and relieved by rest. The feet initially become cold, cyanotic, and numb when exposed to low temperatures; they later redden, tingle, and become hot. The disease's cause is unknown, but it typically affects young male cigarette smokers. Complications include ulceration and gangrene caused by ischemia.

3 Correct answer—**A**

Intermittent claudication—leg pain resulting from muscular activity without adequate oxygen—becomes evident after similar amounts of exertion and is relieved after shorts period of rest. Claudication does not involve ulcers, which develop as a result of a constant reduction of oxygen and nutrients to tissue. It does not occur during rest; rest pain usually indicates impending necrosis or gangrene. Claudication usually is not described as a burning or cold sensation and is not relieved by elevating the legs.

4 Correct answer—**B**

Intermittent claudication typically is the first symptom of arterial insufficiency. It is not associated with phlebitis, venous insufficiency, or mitral regurgitation.

5 Correct answer—D

In the most widely used pulse scale, an absent pulse is indicated by 0; markedly impaired, by 1+; moderately impaired, by 2+; slightly impaired, by 3+; and normal, by 4+. With an abnormal pulse, the amplitude (such as weak, thready, or bounding) also is described. The term *bilateral* indicates that pulses are equal.

6 Correct answer—A

Bruits are abnormal sounds caused by turbulent blood flow through stenotic (partially occluded) blood vessels. Bruits are not associated with occluded blood vessels, hypotension, or collateral circulation.

7 Correct answer—B

Impedence plethysmography (IPG) measures venous outflow; reduced outflow in a patient with calf pain usually indicates deep vein thrombosis. IPG does not detect obstruction of arterial inflow, although this may influence the results. IPG also does not detect distal aneurysms or arteriosclerosis obliterans, both of which are associated with the arterial system.

8 Correct answer—C

Frequent leg movements and exercises increase venous return from the legs. Avoiding ambulation causes venous stasis, increasing the risk of thrombosis. Hyperflexion of the knees interferes with venous return by compressing blood vessels. The proper use of support stockings increases venous return by applying even pressure on superficial veins.

9 Correct answer—A

A heating pad should never be applied to the feet of a patient with compromised arterial supply to the legs; tissue injury may occur before the patient feels any symptoms of it because of impaired sensations. Also, tissue demand for oxygen increases with heat; because the oxygen supply is already inadequate, applying heat may cause necrosis. The other measures are appropriate. Exercise stimulates skeletal muscle contraction, increasing venous return. Warm socks and higher room temperature help keep the patient's feet warm without the risk of tissue damage.

10 Correct answer—D

Raynaud's disease usually occurs in women ages 16 to 40, not older men. Intermittent constriction of cutaneous blood vessels, precipitated by exposure to cold or by emotional stress, produces cyanosis and pallor of the fingers or toes; reactive hyperemia after vasoconstriction causes redness.

11 Correct answer—B

Although the abdominal aortic aneurysm is not always palpable, a pulsatile abdominal mass is an expected finding. Detection depends on the size of the aneurysm as well as the nurse's physical examination skills. Tachycardia, paresis of the legs, and carotid bruits are not caused by an abdominal aortic aneurysm; therefore, they are not expected findings for a patient with this diagnosis.

12 Correct answer—B

Rupture of the aneurysm may cause hypovolemia and can be fatal. Embolism in the foot is a possible complication, but it does not endanger the patient as seriously as rupture does. Cerebrovascular accident and myocardial infarction (MI) are not complications of abdominal aortic aneurysm.

13 Correct answer—D

The dorsalis pedis pulse is located on the top surface of the foot. The popliteal pulse is located behind the knee; the posterior tibial pulse, behind and slightly below the malleolus of the ankle; and the femoral pulse, in the inguinal area.

14 Correct answer—C

Gangrene of the toes indicates irreversible damage, the most severe degree of ischemia caused by arteriosclerosis obliterans. Rest pain, trophic changes (such as changes in color, temperature, nails, and hair distribution), and disabling claudication indicate less severe ischemia.

15 Correct answer—B

In arteriosclerosis obliterans, plaque forms on the wall of an artery. Continuing plaque formation causes partial or complete occlusion as well as loss of vessel wall elasticity; as a result, the artery transports less blood. Symptoms develop when blood flow to a particular area is insufficient; severe symptoms occur when the disease progressively affects more vessels, particularly larger ones.

16 Correct answer—C

The patient with arteriosclerosis obliterans should walk regularly. Walking increases exercise tolerance and may increase collateral circulation. By stating that he has stopped smoking, practices meticulous foot care, and wants to lose weight, the patient shows he understands the disease and the measures to avoid or delay complications.

17 Correct answer—C

Leg measurements should not be taken with the patient standing because it encourages edema, reducing the accuracy of measurements. The dorsal recumbent position prevents edema. Using a felt-tipped pen to mark the measuring tape's position on the leg helps maintain accuracy with subsequent measurements. Bilateral measurements allow comparison between both legs.

18 Correct answer—A

Calf pain is the most likely symptom of thrombophlebitis; the thrombus impedes blood flow, causing inflammation and swelling. Bilateral ankle edema does not occur unless thrombophlebitis affects both legs. The other choices are not manifestations of thrombophlebitis. Foot drop occurs when nerve stimuli to muscles in the foot are interrupted; varicose veins result from abnormal dilation caused by venous valve incompetency.

19 Correct answer—B

Massaging the affected leg may dislodge the thrombus, which might be carried by the blood and forced into a smaller vessel, impeding blood flow (embolism). Maintaining bed rest helps prevent dislodging the thrombus. Elevating the legs on pillows helps reduce edema of the lower extremities by decreasing the force of gravity and improving venous return. Fluid helps reduce blood viscosity, preventing further thrombus formation.

20 Correct answer—A

Shortness of breath is the initial presenting symptom of pulmonary embolism, a serious and potentially life-threatening complication of deep vein thrombosis. Increased skin temperature of the affected leg, calf tenderness, and reddened skin are expected findings of thrombophlebitis that do not require immediate action.

21 Correct answer—C

Support stockings should be applied in the morning before ambulation, when edema is decreased. Most physicians advise their patients to remove the stockings in the evening before sleeping. They should be removed once a day to allow for hygiene, to check the condition of the skin, and to prevent areas of excessive pressure from developing. They should never be rolled down; this causes a tourniquet effect, producing venous stasis rather than preventing it.

22 Correct answer—C

Congestive heart failure (CHF) increases systemic venous pressure, causing distended neck veins. Increased blood volume in the venous system changes capillary membrane permeability, allowing plasma to enter interstitial tissues; this leads to dependent pitting edema. Crushing chest pain unrelieved by rest or nitroglycerin and diaphoresis with cool, clammy skin are common symptoms of MI secondary to coronary artery occlusion. Fever and an elevated white blood cell count are common signs of pericarditis.

23 Correct answer—B

In left ventricular failure, the left ventricle cannot pump the necessary volume of oxygenated blood coming from the lungs, resulting in lung congestion. An upright position allows full chest expansion, which helps relieve dyspnea. The dorsal recumbent position decreases ventilation; elevating the feet increases blood flow to the heart, putting a greater work load on it. The low-Fowler's position with elevated knees may cause pooling of blood in the abdominal area, which may lead to increased ascites and poor diaphragmatic contractions. The left lateral Sims' position has not been proven more effective in emptying to the right side of the heart; besides, an increase in the amount of blood pumped from the right ventricle into the pulmonary circulation would only worsen the patient's condition.

24 Correct answer—A

Chlorothiazide (Diuril) is a diuretic that acts on the distal tubules to increase the excretion of water, sodium, chloride, and potassium; this lowers the circulatory volume and alleviates the patient's symptoms. Digoxin (Lanoxin), not chlorothiazide, strengthens the force of ventricular contraction and slows the heart rate. Chlorothiazide does not affect the metabolic rate.

25 Correct answer—C

This meal is low in sodium, has an item high in potassium (banana), and includes foods from all four basic groups. Bologna, carrot sticks, tuna fish, and celery sticks all have a high sodium content; coffee and tea provide no nutrition.

26 Correct answer—D

Abdominal distention, weakness, paralysis, apathy, depression, and hallucinations are signs of potassium and calcium overdose, not digoxin toxicity. Bradycardia, tachycardia, bigeminy, ectopic beats, and pulse deficits are cardiovascular symptoms of digoxin toxicity. Anorexia, nausea and vomiting, diarrhea, and abdominal pain are GI symptoms of digoxin toxicity. Headache, double or blurred vision, drowsiness, confusion, restlessness, and muscle weakness are neurologic symptoms of digoxin toxicity.

27 Correct answer—A

The sudden cessation of antihypertensive therapy in a patient with moderate to severe hypertension commonly causes hypertensive crisis, resulting in severe arteriolar vasoconstriction in the kidneys. Damaged blood vessels in the renal glomeruli and spasm of the afferent arterioles cause leakage of protein and red blood cells (RBCs) into the urine. The blood urea nitrogen and creatinine levels rise after this acute reduction in renal function. Hyperglycemia is not a characteristic finding with hypertensive crisis. Movement of RBCs through constricted arterioles under pressure traumatizes them, making them appear fragmented on examination.

28 Correct answer—B

The headache, decreased level of consciousness, and unequal pupils are signs and symptoms of hypertensive encephalopathy; they are brought on by increased vascular resistance associated with hypertensive crisis, which leads to cerebral ischemia and edema. The most common adverse effect of antihypertensive medications is hypotension, not hypertension. Thromboembolism may result from hypertensive crisis, but the patient would have diminished or absent peripheral pulses as well as numbness or pain in his extremities. Hypertensive crisis may cause an aneurysm to rupture, but the blood pressure would be significantly reduced.

29 Correct answer—**C**

Smoking elevates blood pressure and increases heart rate; the nurse should encourage the patient to quit smoking and suggest other activities to help him relax. Helping him identify ways to incorporate treatments into his life-style helps prevent the noncompliance associated with complicated treatment plans. Participation in support groups usually increases compliance in patients with a chronic disease. The hospitalized patient may be anxious and distracted, particularly if he is elderly; written instructions can improve compliance by reminding the patient of instructions he has forgotten since discharge.

30 Correct answer—**B**

Elevating the head of the bed reduces cardiac work load; a calm, restful environment helps decrease the anxiety associated with shortness of breath. Positioning the patient flat in bed increases cardiac work load. Elevating the knees reduces venous flow by causing pressure against the popliteal area. Valsalva's maneuver (straining during bowel movements, bending at the waist, or holding the breath while moving) and positioning the patient flat with elevated knees raises intrathoracic pressure, increasing cardiac work load.

31 Correct answer—**D**

Loop diuretics, such as furosemide (Lasix), increase potassium excretion, resulting in hypokalemia in about half the patients taking them. When administering a loop diuretic with digoxin (Lanoxin), the nurse must assess the patient for hypokalemia because arrhythmias—an adverse effect of digoxin—are more likely when the serum potassium level is low. Loop diuretics also cause low, not high, sodium levels. High, not low, uric acid levels may cause gout if the patient's renal function is impaired, which is not indicated in this case. Serum low-density lipoprotein, cholesterol, and triglyceride levels may rise in a patient taking a thiazide diuretic, not a loop diuretic.

32 Correct answer—**C**

Hypertension is a lifelong disease; the patient must understand that she needs to take medication every day to control it. (If hypertension is mild, proper diet, exercise, and weight loss may enable the patient to reduce or stop medication; however, the patient should not try this unless instructed by the physician.) The diet of a patient on diuretic therapy should include foods high in potassium, such as tomatoes, oranges, and bananas. Aerobic exercise (such as walking, swimming, and biking) benefits the cardiovascular system; the patient should avoid anaerobic exercise, such as weight lifting, which may cause severe elevation in both systolic and diastolic blood pressures. Canned and frozen foods are high in sodium, which increase fluid retention and blood pressure; the patient should eat fresh foods instead.

33 Correct answer—D

Malignant hypertension—rapid progression of primary or secondary hypertension—commonly is treated with a potent vasodilator and a loop diuretic. Nitroprusside (Nipride), the vasodilator of choice, can be titrated for rapid pressure reduction when monitoring is available; diazoxide (Hyperstat), which acts directly on the peripheral arteriolar smooth muscle, may be given instead. Treatment must include a loop diuretic, usually furosemide. These drugs are given I.V.; their onset of action is extremely fast. Angiotensin converting enzyme (ACE) inhibitors (which reduce peripheral arterial resistance without affecting heart rate or cardiac work load) and alpha-adrenergic blockers (which block peripheral vascular adrenergic receptors and cause vessel wall relaxation, resulting in peripheral vasodilation) as well as beta-adrenergic blockers (which decrease sympathetic stimulation and renin secretion by the kidneys) may be used to treat primary or essential hypertension but not a medical emergency like malignant hypertension.

34 Correct answer—C

Mitral valve stenosis, which commonly results from rheumatic fever, is caused by stiffening and fusing of the valve leaflets. The chordae tendineae become shorter and thicker, further preventing the valve from opening normally. Valvular atrophy, fibrous ring formation, and valve leaflet widening do not occur in this disease.

35 Correct answer—C

S_2 is the sound made by the closing of the aortic and pulmonary semilunar valves; mitral valve stenosis does not cause this sound to increase. A loud S_1 is commonly heard with mitral valve stenosis; because the mitral valve leaflets are rigid, they increase the intensity of the first heart sound. Adventitious lung sounds and peripheral edema may indicate CHF secondary to ineffective pumping, a result of mitral valve stenosis.

36 Correct answer—A

Intractable vomiting indicates a GI disturbance, which is not a complication of subacute bacterial endocarditis (SBE). Common complications of SBE include spleen involvement, indicated by left upper quadrant pain; kidney involvement, indicated by hematuria; and embolism, indicated by decreasing blood pressure.

37 Correct answer—**A**

Unless complications are present, the patient with SBE does not require complete bed rest after discharge. Antibiotic therapy must be continued for 4 to 6 weeks to prevent relapse. Because endocarditis may be precipitated by minor intrusive procedures, such as dental work and gynecologic examinations, the patient should inform all health care providers beforehand of her condition and request prophylactic antibiotics to prevent relapse of SBE. Signs and symptoms of relapse may be vague and resemble influenza; the patient must recognize them promptly and seek antibiotic treatment to decrease valve damage and complications.

38 Correct answer—**A**

All of these findings are major coronary risk factors. However, a family history of heart disease represents the greatest risk because heredity cannot be changed. Smoking, sedentary life-style, and stressful work environment are factors that can be changed or controlled to reduce the risk of heart disease.

39 Correct answer—**B**

The radioactive thallium rapidly enters viable, well-perfused myocardial tissue, distinguishing it from tissue with poor blood flow or damaged cells. This is an invasive procedure, requiring an I.V. line for thallium infusion. A thallium scan performed during exercise is not a resting scan, nor would it determine coronary artery insufficiency. Cardiac catheterization, another test used in diagnosing heart disease, does not provide the same information as a thallium scan; the scan may provide enough information to make catheterization unnecessary, but catheterization may be necessary to evaluate the extent of coronary artery disease.

40 Correct answer—**B**

Angina pectoris is not always localized in one or two areas. Because pain receptors vary in their responses to ischemic episodes and pain can be referred, angina may be experienced in the chest, epigastrium, neck, either arm or hand, and jaw. Periods of coronary insufficiency cause angina, which usually lasts less than 10 minutes. Angina is relieved by rest, which decreases the demand for oxygen, and by nitroglycerin (Nitro-Bid), which increases the oxygen supply by dilating blood vessels and improving myocardial blood flow.

41 Correct answer—A

All three drugs improve myocardial circulation by increasing blood flow through the coronary arterial system. Diltiazem (Cardizem), a calcium channel blocker, dilates coronary arteries, reduces coronary spasm, decreases arrhythmias by slowing sinoatrial and atrioventricular conduction, and dilates peripheral vasculature to lower arterial blood pressure; isosorbide dinitrate (Isordil) and nitroglycerin, both nitrates, cause arterial and venous dilation. These nitrates must be stored in a dark glass container; metal or plastic containers as well as light cause the drugs to break down and lose their potency. These drugs can help prevent the frequency, intensity, and duration of angina, but they will not eliminate it or cure the condition that causes it. Sublingual nitroglycerin as needed (p.r.n.) relieves chest pain; the drug is administered I.V. to control hypertension associated with surgery.

42 Correct answer—D

By starting oxygen, the nurse improves the patient's arterial oxygen saturation, supplying the myocardium with needed oxygen to minimize tissue damage caused by ischemia. Most emergency departments (EDs) allow the nurse to begin oxygen without a physician's order, and 2 liters/minute is a safe flow rate even for a patient with pulmonary disease. Although the patient may need morphine, the nurse cannot administer it—or start any I.V. lines—without a physician's order. Checking arterial blood gas levels may help in diagnosing the patient's problem but will not help relieve his discomfort. Guided imagery can be beneficial in relieving anxiety and pain, but the nurse must relieve the patient's initial pain and establish a trusting relationship with him before imagery is useful.

43 Correct answer—D

In an acute myocardial infarction (MI), the ST segment and T waves are elevated in the leads for the area in which the MI occurs. The T waves typically invert 4 to 6 hours after an MI, which corresponds with the patient's admission data. Premature ventricular contractions (PVCs) commonly occur with ischemia but do not indicate MI. Q waves typically do not appear for several days after the onset of chest pain and usually are permanent; therefore, they probably indicate a previous MI. ST-segment depression indicates ischemia, not MI.

44 Correct answer—A

Irreversible injury to myocardial tissue produces the MB isoenzyme of creatine phosphokinase (CPK-MB); an elevated CPK-MB level within 2 to 4 hours of the onset of chest pain is the most accurate confirmation of MI. Lactate dehydrogenase and aspartate aminotransferase (formerly serum glutamic-oxaloacetic transaminase) levels as well as erythrocyte sedimentation rate may increase in many other conditions, such as infections, muscle injury, and liver and pulmonary disease.

45 Correct answer—C

Because malignant PVCs fall on or near the T wave, this condition is often called the R-on-T phenomenon. The T wave represents the electrical repolarization (resting phase) of the myocardium, when the heart is most vulnerable to irritable impulses. Any stimulus during this phase, such as a PVC, could cause the ventricle to begin firing in rapid succession—a life-threatening arrhythmia called ventricular tachycardia. The other responses, which do not lead to a dangerous situation, are not characteristics of malignant PVCs.

46 Correct answer—C

Typically, a patient experiences denial in the first 24 hours after MI. He denies the cause and seriousness of the problem, especially after he begins to feel better. The patient may delay seeking treatment; this delay may result in sudden cardiac death outside the hospital. Bargaining and depression are two other stages of grief the patient experiences before acceptance, the final stage.

47 Correct answer—D

Because the contrast medium used during the procedure contains iodine, the nurse must determine if Mr. J. has experienced allergic responses to any iodine preparation or seafood. Heparin is contraindicated because anticoagulation can lead to excessive bleeding during the procedure. A left-sided retrograde cardiac catheterization involves the femoral or brachial artery, not the femoral vein. The physician usually orders nothing-by-mouth status for only 8 to 12 hours before this procedure.

48 Correct answer—C

Pain in the distal, left lower extremity more likely indicates embolism; it is not characteristic of cardiogenic shock. Disorientation,

narrow pulse pressure and thready pulse, and ST-segment elevations in leads II, III and aV_F are manifestations of cardiogenic shock.

49 Correct answer—A

A heart rate under 60 beats/minute indicates bradycardia. The PR
interval normally is 0.12 to 0.20 second; a prolonged interval of 0.26
second indicates atrioventricular (AV) block rather than a normal
sinus rhythm. Because the atrial and ventricular rates are the same,
with no lost or dropped beats, the AV block is first-degree rather
than second-degree or complete heart block.

50 Correct answer—A

The Holter monitor, worn on the patient's belt, records heart activity on tape for a prescribed period; the patient keeps a diary of her
activities and any associated symptoms for the same period. The
tape is later analyzed and correlated with the patient's activities to
help in diagnosing heart problems. The other choices describe
treadmill stress testing, echocardiography or phonocardiography,
and thallium myocardial scanning, respectively.

51 Correct answer—D

Vigorous arm and shoulder movements are restricted for about 6
weeks after permanent pacemaker insertion to prevent dislodging
the electrodes and to allow the incision to heal. After this period, the
patient usually can resume normal activities. No activities, even
heavy lifting, are restricted as long as 6 months; such activities as
needlework are not restricted at all. Pacemakers and their insertion
have little effect on collateral circulation, and patients Mrs. S.'s age
should get mild to moderate exercise, such as by walking.

52 Correct answer—B

This statement indicates a lack of understanding about the signs of
inflammation and possible infection. The patient should report any
signs and symptoms of inflammation at the incision site, such as
fever, discharge, tenderness, and redness. Taking and recording
the pulse daily, obtaining a medical alert bracelet, and avoiding
older, dangerous microwave ovens are proper patient actions.

53 Correct answer—B

Prinzmetal's variant angina is chest pain that occurs during rest. Unresponsive chest pain is called intractable angina; chest pain that occurs in paroxysms while reclining is angina decubitus; and chest
pain during the night is nocturnal angina.

54 Correct answer—**D**

This statement shows that the patient understands the disease and his prognosis. Proper medication, diet, and exercise to promote collateral circulation help slow the progress of inoperable coronary disease; the patient could have many more productive years. Statements about not living long and having to take early retirement indicate incomplete understanding of the disease and diagnosis. Statements about physicians who can cure this type of disease show false hope for a miracle cure.

55 Correct answer—**D**

This response warns the patient that sex may cause chest pain, then provides therapeutic information he can use to prevent pain; this helps the patient make an informed decision. The other three responses do not provide the client with any therapeutic information.

56 Correct answer—**C**

A subendocardial MI may extend and involve larger areas of the myocardium; however, it is considered a relatively mild MI and does not carry a poor prognosis. An inferior epicardial MI involves a small portion of the inferior outer layer of heart muscle; a transmural MI involves the entire thickness of the myocardium.

57 Correct answer—**C**

A third heart sound (S_3) is the first objective sign of left ventricular failure. Crackles and cough and pink, frothy sputum are late signs, signifying congestion from heart failure and pulmonary edema. A fourth heart sound (S_4) is not a sign of left ventricular failure.

58 Correct answer—**B**

Dopamine, a peripheral vasopressor, and nitroprusside (Nipride), a vasodilator, sometimes are used together to maintain blood pressure within a given range and to dilate coronary blood vessels, which improves left ventricular function and cardiac output. These two drugs are not incompatible. They do not cause localized pain unless extravasation occurs. To reduce the risk of dopamine extravasation, which causes severe tissue destruction, the nurse should administer the drug through a large vein in the antecubital fossa rather than a small one in the hand. Nitroprusside should never be piggybacked with another I.V. drug and administered through a single site; the nurse must infuse the drug separately and monitor the patient continuously for possible adverse reaction.

CHAPTER 3

Neurosensory System

Questions

1 Which medication is *not* appropriate for a postoperative patient with a craniotomy?

A. Dexamethasone (Decadron)
B. Phenytoin (Dilantin)
C. Codeine
D. Meperidine (Demerol)

2 Which type of brain tumor is most common in adults?

A. Glioma
B. Meningioma
C. Metastatic tumor
D. Congenital tumor

3 All of the following signs indicate increased intracranial pressure (ICP) *except:*

A. Papilledema
B. Decreased level of consciousness
C. Tachycardia
D. Vomiting

4 Cerebral perfusion pressure, which is closely related to blood flow, is equal to:

A. ICP minus mean arterial pressure (MAP)
B. The difference between diastolic and systolic blood pressures minus ICP
C. MAP minus ICP
D. MAP plus ICP

5 Which nursing activity does *not* reduce or prevent an increase in ICP?

A. Elevating the head of the bed 30 degrees
B. Suctioning every 2 hours to maintain a patent airway
C. Teaching the patient not to strain during bowel movements
D. Providing respiratory care to prevent hypercapnia and hypoxia

6 Lower motor neuron disease may cause various abnormal movements. Discrete, jerky, purposeless movement seen in the distal extremities and face is called:

A. Athetosis
B. Dystonia
C. Chorea
D. Myoclonus

7 Which measure should the nurse use to help a blind patient ambulate?

A. Steer the patient from behind while telling him what is ahead
B. Encourage the patient to count steps while shuffling his feet
C. Allow the patient to follow behind the nurse while lightly holding her elbow
D. Hold the patient's hand and encourage him to walk at a brisk pace

8 Which assessment finding most strongly indicates Ménière's disease?

A. Nausea
B. Tinnitus
C. Vertigo
D. Neurosensory hearing loss

9 To reduce dizziness and prevent falling in a patient with Ménière's disease, the nurse should take all of the following measures *except:*

A. Raising the bed's side rails
B. Having the patient close his eyes when lying down
C. Allowing the patient to assume a comfortable position
D. Administering a diuretic as ordered

10 Before an ophthalmologic examination, the physician commonly instills atropine sulfate (Isopto Atropine) 1% eye drops to:

A. Prevent adhesions
B. Increase vitreous humor flow
C. Dilate the pupils
D. Decrease intraocular pressure

11 All of the following clinical manifestations are characteristic of retinal detachment *except:*

A. Blurred vision
B. Dull eye pain
C. Spots floating before the eyes
D. Flashes of light

SITUATION

L., a 20-year-old female student, is admitted to the hospital with seizures.

Questions 12 to 16 refer to this situation.

12 Which procedure helps diagnose the type of seizure?

A. Echocardiography
B. Electrocardiography
C. Electroencephalography
D. Endarterectomy

13 L. states, "I see flickering lights right before I have a seizure." This phenomenon is known as:

A. Postictal state
B. Aura
C. Tonic phase
D. Clonic phase

14 L. is to be discharged on phenytoin therapy. When teaching L. about her medication, the nurse should:

A. Instruct her to take the drug on an empty stomach
B. Instruct her to avoid massaging her gums, since massage can precipitate bleeding
C. Warn her not to stop taking her medication without medical supervision
D. Instruct her to undergo complete blood count testing annually

15 After the patient-teaching session on drug therapy, the nurse observes that L. is quiet and withdrawn. When the nurse asks why, L. says, "I feel so different—will I ever fit in?" The most appropriate response by the nurse would be:

A. "You feel different?"
B. "No, your condition will always make you feel different"
C. "Taking your medication will make you feel more normal"
D. "Everyone your age feels that way"

16 L. continues undergoing extensive health teaching about her condition. Which behavior would indicate to the nurse that she understands her condition and any necessary life-style changes?

A. Avoiding physical activity
B. Swimming 30 minutes a day by herself
C. Taking her medication only when she feels dizzy
D. Wearing a medical alert bracelet

SITUATION

Mr. J., a 65-year-old retired assembly-line worker, is admitted to the hospital with a diagnosis of Parkinson's disease.

Questions 17 to 21 refer to this situation.

17 Which clinical features of the disease should the nurse expect to observe during admission assessment?

A. Muscle flaccidity and lethargy
B. Masklike face and shuffling gait
C. Dry skin and drooling
D. Swayback stance and muscle cramps

18 Mr. J.'s symptoms are caused by:

A. Cerebral anoxia
B. Congenital abnormalities in neuronal transmission in the brain
C. An imbalance in dopamine and acetylcholine levels
D. An imbalance in glucose and adenosine triphosphate levels

19 The physician orders 1 mg of benztropine mesylate (Cogentin) P.O. daily for Mr. J. Which finding suggests a favorable effect from this medication?

A. Decreased muscle rigidity
B. Decreased tremors
C. Decreased dizziness
D. Decreased confusion

20 The most important nursing action during Mr. J.'s hospitalization is:

A. Scheduling routine home visits by the community health nurse
B. Scheduling daily sessions with the speech therapist
C. Discontinuing all over-the-counter medications
D. Maintaining a daily exercise program

21 The physician adds levodopa (Larodopa) to Mr. J.'s drug regimen. Which precaution should the nurse give Mr. J. during the patient-teaching session before discharge?

A. "Take a vitamin B$_6$ tablet with each dose of levodopa"
B. "Eat high-protein meals"
C. "Wear elastic stockings to help avoid orthostatic hypotension"
D. "Take levodopa only on an empty stomach"

SITUATION

Mr. M., a 55-year-old tailor, is admitted to the hospital, complaining of difficulty holding objects. He states that his condition has progressively worsened. The physician suspects amyotrophic lateral sclerosis (ALS).

Questions 22 to 24 refer to this situation.

22 Which procedure confirms a diagnosis of ALS?

A. Creatine phosphokinase (CPK) test
B. Skeletal muscle biopsy
C. Lumbar puncture
D. Romberg test

23 Characteristic clinical manifestations of ALS do *not* include:

A. Loss of bowel and urine control
B. Uncontrolled outbursts of crying
C. Aphagia and dysarthria
D. Fasciculation of the involved muscles

24 After testing confirms the diagnosis of ALS, the nurse prepares Mr. M. for discharge. The patient-teaching session should cover all of the following topics *except:*

A. Avoiding fatigue and extreme cold
B. Wearing well-fitting, supportive shoes
C. Using diaphragmatic breathing techniques
D. Adhering to a low-residue diet

SITUATION

Mrs. G., a 23-year-old secretary, is admitted to the hospital because of extreme muscle fatigue on exertion. Her physician suspects myasthenia gravis.

Questions 25 to 28 refer to this situation.

25 Which test is most reliable in confirming a diagnosis of myasthenia gravis?

A. Stress test
B. Edrophonium (Tensilon) test
C. Glucose tolerance test
D. Sweat chloride test

26 Which assessment findings are most likely in a patient with myasthenia gravis?

A. Restlessness, decreased level of consciousness, and a history of extreme muscle weakness in the morning
B. Unequal pupillary response, diplopia, and inability to hold her mouth closed
C. Frequent changes in facial expression, exophthalmos, and a low-pitched voice
D. Ptosis, dysphagia, and a soft, nasal voice

27 While providing morning care, the nurse observes that Mrs. G. is wheezing and pale with a respiratory rate of 40 breaths/minute. The nurse should:

A. Notify the physician immediately
B. Administer oxygen at 2 liters/minute via nasal cannula
C. Administer 500 mg of aminophylline (Aminophyllin) I.V.
D. Have the patient cough and deep breathe every 2 hours

28 The nurse administers neostigmine (Prostigmin) to Mrs. G. Possible favorable results include:

A. Increased self-care activity and decreased dysphagia
B. Increased white blood cell count and improved memory
C. Improved pupillary and tactile stimulation responses
D. Mild sedative effects without "hangover" symptoms

SITUATION

Mrs. K., a 75-year-old widow with Alzheimer's disease, is brought to the emergency department (ED) by her daughter after falling at an adult care center. Her injuries appear to be minor, but the center requested a medical evaluation. Mrs. K. has lived with her daughter, son-in-law, and two grandchildren for the past 3 years because her physician advised her that she could no longer live alone.

Questions 29 to 32 refer to this situation.

29 While Mrs. K.'s injuries are being assessed, her daughter tells the nurse that Mrs. K. is prone to irrational and often violent outbursts, which are becoming more frequent. She asks what causes these outbursts. The nurse should respond that they are caused by:

A. Inadequate exercise
B. Forgetfulness
C. Sensory overload
D. Prolonged sleep

30 Which nursing intervention is most important for Mrs. K.?

A. Halting the deterioration process
B. Providing a safe environment
C. Keeping her quiet
D. Teaching good personal hygiene habits

31 Alzheimer's disease is diagnosed definitively through:

A. Computed tomography scanning
B. A history of dementia
C. Autopsy
D. Neuropsychological testing

32 Medical-pharmacologic management of Alzheimer's disease is aimed at controlling:

A. Abnormal protein in the brain
B. Undesirable symptoms
C. Environmental toxins
D. Urinary incontinence

SITUATION

Mrs. J., a 43-year-old schoolteacher, is admitted to the unit with symmetrical weakness of her lower extremities. After testing, the physician diagnoses Guillain-Barré syndrome.

Questions 33 to 36 refer to this situation.

33 The cause of Guillain-Barré syndrome is:

A. A postoperative complication
B. A respiratory infection
C. Gastroenteritis
D. Unknown

34 The pathophysiologic mechanism of Guillain-Barré syndrome is:

A. Demyelination and degeneration of the myelin sheath
B. Pigmented neuron loss
C. Defective impulse transmission between nerve and muscle cells
D. An unexplained loss of basal ganglia cells

35 Routine assessment for Mrs. J. should include checking for:

A. Impaired gag and swallowing reflexes
B. Ptosis
C. Impaired hearing
D. Facial twitching

36 Which outcome is most likely for Mrs. J.?

A. Frequent exacerbations
B. Death
C. Chronic infections
D. Slow but complete recovery

SITUATION

N., a 21-year-old college student, is brought to the ED after sustaining a gunshot wound to the neck. His condition was stabilized at the scene of the shooting by emergency medical technicians. He is conscious with a blood pressure of 90/60 mm Hg, a pulse rate of 56 beats/minute, and a respiratory rate of 14 breaths/minute. The trauma team ascertains that N. is suffering from spinal shock.

Questions 37 to 39 refer to this situation.

---

37 The physician determines that N. has a transection of the spinal cord at level C5. This type of injury causes:

A. Decreased respiratory function
B. No change in respiratory function
C. Loss of respiratory function
D. Transient changes in respiratory function

---

38 Various types of beds and frames are used for patients with spinal cord injuries. The one that prevents pressure ulcers, cardiopulmonary complications, muscle wasting, and urinary stasis and calculi through continuous side-to-side motion is the:

A. Air-fluidized (Clinitron) bed
B. Wedge (Stryker) frame
C. Circular electric (CircOlectric) bed
D. Kinetic therapy (Roto Rest) bed

---

39 When assessing N. for stress ulcers caused by excessive release of hydrochloric acid in the stomach, the nurse may note all of the following manifestations *except:*

A. Expanding abdominal girth
B. Abdominal pain and tenderness
C. Melena
D. A gradual drop in hematocrit

SITUATION

Mrs. S., a 32-year-old homemaker, is admitted to the hospital with a history of urine retention. Her physician suspects multiple sclerosis (MS).

Questions 40 to 45 refer to this situation.

40 Which diagnostic tool helps confirm a diagnosis of MS?

A. Cerebrospinal fluid analysis
B. Skull X-rays
C. Electroencephalography
D. Electromyography

41 During the nurse's assessment, Mrs. S. states that she has experienced some spastic weakness of her lower extremities. This weakness is caused by:

A. Areas of demyelination in the main motor pathways of the spinal cord
B. Degeneration of nerve cells in the extrapyramidal system
C. Sudden, excessive discharge from cerebral neurons
D. Dilation of the walls of a cerebral artery

42 While obtaining a history from Mrs. S., the nurse notices an involuntary, rhythmic, and rapid jerking of the eyeballs when Mrs. S. looks to the side. This is called:

A. Diplopia
B. Nystagmus
C. Hemianopia
D. Esophoria

43 Mrs. S.'s physician orders a myelogram using a water-soluble contrast medium. Which nursing activity is most appropriate for Mrs. S. after this procedure?

A. Restricting fluids for 6 to 10 hours
B. Monitoring level of consciousness
C. Elevating the head of the bed 15 to 30 degrees
D. Placing the patient in a recumbent position for 12 to 24 hours

44 The physician orders baclofen (Lioresal) therapy to reduce muscle spasm as well as urinary self-catheterization every 4 hours. Which instruction should the nurse give Mrs. S. about the medication?

A. "Take it on an empty stomach"
B. "Take it only when symptoms are present"
C. "Do not discontinue it abruptly"
D. "Discontinue it if your urine output increases"

45 During the patient-teaching session, the nurse tells Mrs. S. that following the self-catheterization schedule should:

A. Promote independence
B. Prevent urinary tract infections
C. Permit more normal sexual relations
D. Preserve bladder tone

SITUATION

Mr. W., a 66-year-old retired fireman, is brought to the ED by ambulance after his wife had difficulty waking him in the morning. Mrs. W. states that her husband is having difficulty moving the right side of his body and "doesn't seem to be himself." Physical examination reveals Mr. W. has right-sided hemiplegia and a communication problem. The physician diagnoses a cerebrovascular accident of the left cerebral hemisphere.

Questions 46 and 47 refer to this situation.

46 During nursing assessment, Mr. W. speaks in a rambling manner and is unable to repeat words spoken to him. Which area of the brain most likely is affected?

A. Brodmann's area
B. Wernicke's area
C. Broca's area
D. Foramen magnum

47 The long-term goal for Mr. W. should focus on:

A. Rehabilitating the patient
B. Maintaining his respiratory function
C. Providing respite care services for his caregiver
D. Correcting cognitive deficits

SITUATION

Mr. P., a 45-year-old construction worker, developed acute pain in his right eye while at work. He is brought to the ED; after a complete physical examination, the physician diagnoses acute closed-angle glaucoma.

Questions 48 and 49 refer to this situation.

48 Which statement about the clinical manifestations of acute closed-angle glaucoma is *not* correct?

A. Nausea and vomiting usually occur
B. The patient commonly sees rainbows around lights
C. Ocular pain results from increased intracranial pressure
D. The patient's vision becomes cloudy and blurred

49 To confirm the diagnosis, the physician orders tonometry testing for Mr. P. This test:

A. Measures the eyes' ability to focus on close objects
B. Measures intraocular pressure
C. Permits direct visualization of the retina
D. Evaluates the corneal reflex

The physician orders pilocarpine (Isopto Carpine) 1% in Mr. P.'s affected eye and 500 mg of acetazolamide (Diamox) I.V.

Questions 50 to 54 continue the situation.

50 When administering pilocarpine (Isopto Carpine) eye drops to Mr. P., the nurse should:

A. Place a drop in the inner canthus of the eye
B. Tell the patient to squeeze his eyelids after instillation of the drops
C. Instruct him to look to the side when he feels the drop
D. Tilt his head backward and incline it to the right

51 Which physiologic response should the nurse expect after administering pilocarpine?

A. Pupil dilation
B. Diminished lacrimation
C. Decreased intraocular pressure
D. Increased sensitivity to light

52 Which nursing action is most appropriate after administering acetazolamide to Mr. P.?

A. Measuring his urine output
B. Checking his pupillary reaction to light
C. Keeping his room semidarkened
D. Raising his bed's side rails

53 Atropine is contraindicated for Mr. P. because it may:

A. Precipitate an acute attack of glaucoma
B. Overstimulate the lacrimal ducts
C. Induce strong contraction of the ciliary body
D. Cause extreme pupillary contraction

54 The physician schedules a peripheral iridectomy of Mr. P.'s affected eye. The primary purpose of this procedure is to:

A. Prevent blood from entering the anterior chamber of the eye
B. Decrease the production of vitreous humor
C. Enhance the drainage of aqueous humor
D. Permit pupillary dilation

SITUATION

Mrs. S., a 70-year-old widow, has been in fairly good health until recently. Although she has been wearing her prescription eyeglasses, her vision has gradually deteriorated. A thorough ophthalmic examination reveals bilateral cataracts. The physician schedules an extracapsular cataract extraction of the left eye; the same procedure will later be performed on the right eye.

Questions 55 to 60 refer to this situation.

55 A cataract is defined as:

A. An abnormal fold of membrane extending onto the cornea
B. An opacity of the crystalline lens
C. Edema of the optic disk
D. A blind spot in the visual field

56 The function of the lens is to:

A. Transmit visual impulses to the brain
B. Enable light rays to focus on the retina
C. Provide nourishment to the eye
D. Dilate and contract according to light intensity

57 The physican orders cyclopentolate (Cyclogyl) 0.5% eye drops in Mrs. S.'s left eye 2 hours before surgery. The purpose of this medication is to:

A. Promote pupil contraction
B. Increase the production of aqueous humor
C. Increase intraocular pressure
D. Dilate the pupil

58 Immediately before surgery, the physician orders 50 mg of hydroxyzine (Vistaril) I.M. and 35 mg of meperidine (Demerol) I.M. After Mrs. S. receives these medications, the nurse should:

A. Ensure that the patient voids
B. Raise the bed's side rails
C. Check the patient's vital signs
D. Evaluate the patient's pupillary reaction to light

59 Which postoperative finding should the nurse report promptly to the physician?

A. Sudden ocular pain
B. Swelling of the eyelids
C. Hazy vision
D. Slight nausea

60 Before Mrs. S.'s discharge, the nurse must instruct her to:

A. Cough and deep breathe periodically
B. Follow a low-fiber diet
C. Perform eye muscle exercises regularly
D. Wear an eye shield while sleeping

SITUATION

Ms. L., a 34-year-old secretary, comes to the ear clinic complaining of mild nausea, dizziness, and occasional "buzzing" in her right ear. She has a history of allergies and frequent episodes of sinusitis.

Questions 61 and 62 refer to this situation.

61 Which technique would permit better visualization of Ms. L.'s external auditory canal?

A. Pulling the pinna down and back
B. Tilting the head and depressing the tragus
C. Pulling the pinna up and back
D. Holding the otoscope upside-down in the dominant hand

62 Ms. L. has a negative result on the Rinne test. This means she hears the vibrations from a tuning fork:

A. Longer or louder by bone conduction than by air conduction
B. Poorly by both air and bone conduction
C. Longer by air conduction than by bone conduction
D. Equally well by air and bone conduction

Answer sheet

A B C D	A B C D	A B C D
1 ○○○○	31 ○○○○	61 ○○○○
2 ○○○○	32 ○○○○	62 ○○○○
3 ○○○○	33 ○○○○	
4 ○○○○	34 ○○○○	
5 ○○○○	35 ○○○○	
6 ○○○○	36 ○○○○	
7 ○○○○	37 ○○○○	
8 ○○○○	38 ○○○○	
9 ○○○○	39 ○○○○	
10 ○○○○	40 ○○○○	
11 ○○○○	41 ○○○○	
12 ○○○○	42 ○○○○	
13 ○○○○	43 ○○○○	
14 ○○○○	44 ○○○○	
15 ○○○○	45 ○○○○	
16 ○○○○	46 ○○○○	
17 ○○○○	47 ○○○○	
18 ○○○○	48 ○○○○	
19 ○○○○	49 ○○○○	
20 ○○○○	50 ○○○○	
21 ○○○○	51 ○○○○	
22 ○○○○	52 ○○○○	
23 ○○○○	53 ○○○○	
24 ○○○○	54 ○○○○	
25 ○○○○	55 ○○○○	
26 ○○○○	56 ○○○○	
27 ○○○○	57 ○○○○	
28 ○○○○	58 ○○○○	
29 ○○○○	59 ○○○○	
30 ○○○○	60 ○○○○	

Answers and rationales

1 Correct answer—**D**

Meperidine (Demerol) is not given postoperatively to a craniotomy patient because it may mask signs of neurologic problems, such as changes in level of consciousness or abnormal pupillary reactions or size; the drug may also cause respiratory depression. Dexamethasone (Decadron) is given to control cerebral edema. Phenytoin (Dilantin) is given to prevent generalized tonic-clonic seizures. Codeine is used as an analgesic for severe headache; this mild narcotic's activity does not interfere with neurologic assessment.

2 Correct answer—**A**

Gliomas account for almost half of all brain tumors in adults; meningiomas account for approximately 15%, and metastatic and congenital tumors account for less than 10% each. The remainder consists of pituitary adenomas, acoustic neuromas, and blood vessel tumors.

3 Correct answer—**C**

Bradycardia, not tachycardia, accompanied by hypertension is a sign of increased intracranial pressure (ICP). Other signs include nausea and vomiting, decreased level of consciousness, and headache; papilledema is a late sign.

4 Correct answer—**C**

Cerebral perfusion pressure (CPP), which is normally 80 to 90 mm Hg, is determined by subtracting ICP from MAP. A CPP of 50 mm Hg is required for adequate blood flow to the brain. Systolic and diastolic blood pressures are not used to determine CPP.

5 Correct answer—**B**

Suctioning may cause hypoxemia, which leads to increased blood pressure; this may increase ICP by as much as 35 mm Hg. This increase can be prevented in some cases by administering I.V. lidocaine (Xylocaine) before pulmonary suctioning. Although the mechanism is uncertain, lidocaine may block the cough reflex, function as a general anesthetic, or cause cardiovascular depression and thus reduce cerebral blood flow. Elevating the head of the bed increases cerebral venous return, decreasing ICP. Teaching the patient not to strain during bowel movements helps prevent the increased intrathoracic pressure and ICP this can cause. Providing respiratory care is appropriate because hypercapnia and hypoxia cause cerebral vasodilation, which increases cerebral circulating volume and ICP.

---

6 Correct answer—**C**

A discrete, jerky, purposeless movement seen in the distal extremities and face is called chorea. Athetosis is gross, writhing, wormlike movement. Dystonia is prolonged twisting movement. Myoclonus is a sudden muscle contraction of varying intensity, which may involve only a small part of one extremity or the entire body.

---

7 Correct answer—**C**

By walking ahead of the patient at a normal pace, the nurse can identify and eliminate obstacles in the patient's path; allowing the patient to hold the nurse's elbow lightly provides a sense of security without total dependency. Steering the patient from behind while telling him what is ahead provides little physical support for the patient and increases the risk of injury. Counting steps might help the patient judge distances, but shuffling his feet would defeat this purpose. The nurse should never hold the patient's hand and encourage him to walk briskly because a hurried pace increases the risk of injury.

---

8 Correct answer—**C**

The strongest indication of Ménière's disease is vertigo, a sensation of irregular or whirling motion of oneself or of surrounding objects. Nausea commonly accompanies vertigo, but nausea by itself may be caused by many diseases. Tinnitus (a buzzing sound in the ears) and neurosensory hearing loss also occur in Ménière's disease because of cochlear labyrinth disturbances (although hearing loss may not occur early in the disease); however, these findings also could result from other diseases. Vertigo accompanied by tinnitus and neurosensory hearing loss confirms a diagnosis of Ménière's disease.

---

9 Correct answer—**D**

A diuretic will not reduce dizziness or prevent falling in a patient with Ménière's disease. Raising the bed's side rails, having the patient close his eyes when lying down, and allowing him to assume a comfortable position are all appropriate nursing measures.

---

10 Correct answer—**C**

Atropine sulfate (Isopto Atropine) 1% eye drops are instilled before ophthalmologic examination to dilate the pupils; this mydriatic effect allows the physician to readily examine the internal eye structures. Because atropine has a cycloplegic effect as well, it is used postoperatively—not before an examination—to prevent adhesions (synechiae). Atropine does not affect vitreous humor flow or intraocular pressure.

11 Correct answer—B

Because the retina contains no pain-transmitting neuron fibers, pain is not a characteristic clinical manifestation of retinal detachment. Blurred vision, sometimes described as a veil over the eye, is a common complaint; because the retina receives visual images and transmits them to the brain via the optic nerve, most retinal disorders will cause blurred vision. The retina is attached to the choroid, a pigmented layer that contains blood vessels to nourish the retina; floating spots result from pigment or blood cells escaping into the vitreous humor when the retina tears. Flashes of light are caused by vitreous traction on the retina.

12 Correct answer—C

Electroencephalography identifies patterns of electrical activity that can be correlated with particular types of seizures; it localizes an epileptogenic focus (trigger area for seizure activity) in the brain. Echocardiography records the position and motion of the heart walls or internal structures of the heart and neighboring tissue. Electrocardiography provides a tracing representing the heart's electrical activity. Endarterectomy is a surgical procedure in which thickened atheromatous areas are excised from the innermost layer of an artery.

13 Correct answer—B

The aura alerts the patient that a seizure is imminent, allowing her to seek privacy and a safe place to lie down before the seizure begins. The aura may involve visual disturbances, dizziness, numbness, or other sensations that the patient may find difficult to describe exactly. The postictal state is the period of lethargy and confusion the patient experiences after a seizure. A tonic phase is a period of major tonic contraction of the musculature during a seizure. A clonic phase is a period of violent, rhythmic muscular contractions accompanied by strenuous hyperventilation.

14 Correct answer—C

Sudden withdrawal of antiseizure medication can cause an increase in seizure frequency or precipitate status epilepticus. To avoid gastritis, the patient should not take phenytoin on an empty stomach. The patient should brush her teeth frequently and massage her gums to prevent gingival infection. Blood evaluations typically are performed monthly during early therapy and every 6 months during prolonged therapy when the patient is on an antiseizure drug that depresses hemopoiesis, such as phenytoin.

15 Correct answer—A

This response uses the therapeutic communication technique of reflection, which encourages the patient to tell the nurse more about her feelings. Responding that seizures will always make the patient feel different is negative and prevents a trusting nurse-patient relationship. Responding that the medication will help control seizure activity is inappropriate because the lifelong drug therapy may be a factor in the patient's feelings. Responding that everyone her age feels the same way is inappropriate because this ignores the effect of the disease on the patient's psychosocial health.

16 Correct answer—D

A seizure patient should carry a wallet card and wear an appropriate medical alert bracelet. This provides others with necessary information if the patient has a seizure or needs other emergency treatment. Physical and mental activity tends to inhibit, not stimulate, a seizure; the patient should not avoid exercise. However, the patient should avoid swimming alone or engaging in other solitary sports, occupations, or hobbies because of the danger that a seizure will occur with no one nearby to help. Antiseizure medication must be taken daily; the dosage may be adjusted because of recurrent illness, weight changes, or increased stress.

17 Correct answer—B

Parkinson's disease causes rigidity of the facial muscles, resulting in a masklike, staring appearance. Because the disease affects postural reflexes, the patient has difficulty maintaining balance and usually walks in a stooped-over position with small, shuffling steps, commonly accelerating almost to a trot. Muscular rigidity and restlessness, not muscular flaccidity and lethargy, are characteristic of Parkinson's disease. Drooling may result from decreased frequency of swallowing because of facial and pharyngeal muscle rigidity; however, skin usually is not dry but oily, probably from hypothalamic dysfunction, which causes increased sebotropic hormone release. Also, many patients perspire excessively because of a disorder of the hypothalamic heat-regulator mechanism as well as impairment of perspiration controls. Muscle cramps in the legs, neck, and trunk are common, probably because of muscle rigidity; however, difficulty in maintaining balance results in a stooped-over position, not a swayback stance.

18 Correct answer—C

Parkinson's disease results from an imbalance in endogenous dopamine and acetylcholine levels. Normally, dopamine and acetylcholine function interdependently; their opposing actions maintain a balance between excitation and inhibition in the striatum. Parkinson's disease causes a loss of dopaminergic neurons in the substantia nigra and a decreased dopamine supply. This results in a relative increase of acetylcholine activity, producing the symptoms of Parkinson's disease. These symptoms are not caused by hypoxia or by congenital abnormalities. Glucose and adenosine triphosphate are substances associated with skeletal muscle activity.

19 Correct answer—B

Anticholinergics, such as benztropine mesylate (Cogentin), reduce the cholinergic activity caused by decreased dopamine levels and decrease tremors. Muscle rigidity typically is treated with amantadine (Symmetrel) or carbidopa-levodopa (Sinemet). Possible adverse effects of anticholinergic drugs include increased dizziness and confusion; benztropine therapy will not decrease these symptoms.

20 Correct answer—D

For the patient with Parkinson's disease, a daily exercise program, including range-of-motion exercises for all extremities, is essential to maintain physical function. Home visits by a community health nurse may not be necessary unless the patient experiences problems after discharge. A patient on drug therapy usually does not have speech problems. Over-the-counter medications are not given in the hospital; however, the nurse should advise the patient to avoid any cough, cold, or hay fever remedies unless approved by his physician because they contain anticholinergic and antihistamine agents.

21 Correct answer—C

Orthostatic hypotension is a common adverse effect of levodopa therapy. Elastic stockings promote venous return from the extremities; pooling of blood in the extremities can worsen orthostasis. Pyridoxine (vitamin B_6), a cofactor of the enzyme dopa decarboxylase, increases the decarboxylation of levodopa in the liver, thus decreasing the amount that can be converted to dopamine in the brain. Therefore, the patient on levodopa therapy should not take vitamin

B$_6$ or multivitamin preparations that include it. High-protein meals block the effect of levodopa; therefore, the patient should limit his intake of milk, meat, fish, poultry, cheese, eggs, nuts, sunflower seeds, and whole grain and soybean products. The patient should take the drug with meals to decrease nausea, a common adverse effect.

22 Correct answer—B

A skeletal muscle biopsy identifies the presence or absence of degenerative muscle fibers and differentiates between neurogenic and amyotrophic disease. Serum enzymes, such as creatine phosphokinase (CPK), are present in all muscle tissue; an increased level indicates damage but does not confirm the diagnosis. Because the results of a lumbar puncture on a patient with amyotrophic lateral sclerosis (ALS) usually are normal, this procedure is inconclusive. The Romberg test identifies loss of position sense after a cerebral concussion; it does not confirm ALS.

23 Correct answer—A

The patient with ALS usually does not lose urinary and bowel sphincter control because the disease does not affect the spinal nerves controlling these muscles. However, other muscles that control the neck, pharynx, larynx, trunk, and legs atrophy from the gradual degeneration of motor neurons; this can lead to aphagia, dysarthria, uncontrolled outbursts of laughing or crying, and fasciculation of the involved muscles.

24 Correct answer—D

Because muscle atrophy leads to poor peristalsis, the patient is predisposed to constipation; a high-residue diet with a high fiber content helps correct this. The patient should avoid extreme heat, which may cause transient muscle weakness; he should also pace his activities to prevent fatigue. Well-fitting, supportive shoes will help the patient maintain his balance, lessening fatigue. Respiratory dysfunction is a common complication of ALS; diaphragmatic breathing techniques will help maintain or improve respiratory function by training the muscles to work more efficiently.

25 Correct answer—B

The most useful and highly reliable diagnostic test for myasthenia gravis, the edrophonium (Tensilon) test is performed by drawing 10 mg of the drug into a syringe and administering 2 mg I.V. If muscle function does not improve, the remaining 8 mg are injected. Within 30 to 60 seconds of the first dose, most patients with myasthenia gravis will demonstrate marked improvement in muscle tone lasting 4 to 5 minutes; the drug inhibits the destruction of acetylcholine, promoting the transmission of impulses from nerves to muscles. The stress test confirms cardiac ischemia. The glucose tolerance test confirms diabetes mellitus in patients with high-normal or slightly elevated blood glucose levels. The sweat chloride test confirms cystic fibrosis.

26 Correct answer—D

Myasthenia gravis causes weakness in the elevator palpebra muscle, resulting in ptosis. The disease affects the muscles used in chewing, causing dysphagia. It also destroys acetylcholine sites in muscles used in speaking; this weakens muscle contractions, resulting in a soft, nasal voice. The patient may be restless because of respiratory difficulty and anxiety; however, muscle weakness usually worsens in the afternoon and evening, and decreased level of consciousness is not common. Myasthenia gravis may cause diplopia or an inability to hold the mouth closed if it affects the lateral rectus, masseter, medial pterygoid, and temporalis muscles; however, pupillary response remains normal because the disease does not affect the ciliary muscle. Exophthalmos and a low-pitched voice are not common with myasthenia gravis; weakness of the facial muscles typically prevents changes in facial expression.

27 Correct answer—A

Because ineffective breathing pattern and airway clearance are life-threatening complications of myasthenia gravis, the nurse should notify the physician immediately. The disease affects acetylcholine sites at the neuromuscular junctions of the sternocleidomastoid, anterior serratus, scalene, and external intercostal muscles, which prevents complete depolarization of those muscles. This weakens muscular contraction during inspiration, possibly leading to respiratory failure. The physician probably will order arterial blood gas analysis after being notified; the nurse should not administer oxygen beforehand to ensure the accuracy of the results. Aminophylline (Aminophyllin), which relaxes the smooth muscles of the bronchial airways, must be ordered by the physician; it is given only after the patient's status is evaluated and myasthenic and cholinergic crises have been ruled out. Because myasthenia gravis weakens muscular contraction during inspiration, coughing and deep breathing will not improve the patient's respiratory function.

28 Correct answer—A

Neostigmine (Prostigmin), an anticholinesterase medication, prolongs the action of acetylcholine by inhibiting its hydrolysis. This prolonged action allows complete depolarization of skeletal muscle, decreasing the weakness associated with myasthenia gravis. Increased self-care activity and decreased dysphagia are likely results of this decreased weakness. Myasthenia gravis does not cause decreased white blood cell count, memory disturbances, pupillary response deficits, or sensory changes. Sedation is not a common effect of neostigmine.

29 Correct answer—C

Irrational, violent outbursts are caused by sensory overload, such as excessive environmental stimuli, increased stress and an inability to cope, and unfamiliar surroundings. Inadequate exercise and prolonged sleep may lead to sleep pattern disturbances, and forgetfulness may cause self-care deficits, such as inadequate grooming, toileting, and nutrition; however, they do not cause violent outbursts.

30 Correct answer—B

Alzheimer's disease causes physical and mental disabilities, placing Mrs. K. at high risk for accidents and infection; the nurse must provide a safe environment to minimize this risk. No effective treatment exists for the disease or the deterioration it causes. Rather than keep the patient quiet, the nurse should try to prevent her from becoming withdrawn and isolated, which is common in the patient with Alzheimer's disease. Good personal hygiene is desirable but not as important as a safe environment; also, the patient's forgetfulness and regressed behavior may prevent her from learning good hygiene habits.

31 Correct answer—C

Alzheimer's disease can be diagnosed definitively only during autopsy when the presence of neurofibrillary tangles is documented. A computed tomography (CT) scan may show brain atrophy and enlarged ventricles in the later stages of the disease, but these findings may be seen in patients with other diseases and even in healthy individuals. Dementia may be caused by other degenerative diseases of the brain, vascular conditions, tumors, or alcohol or drug toxicity. Neuropsychological testing can help document the degree of cognitive dysfunction, but it does not definitively diagnose Alzheimer's disease.

32 Correct answer—B

The medical-pharmacologic management of Alzheimer's disease is aimed at controlling undesirable symptoms the patient may demonstrate, such as agitation, anxiety, restlessness, and depression. Abnormal protein in the brain is an etiologic factor that cannot be controlled. Environmental toxins and urinary incontinence cannot be controlled through medical-pharmacologic management.

33 Correct answer—D

The precise cause of Guillain-Barré syndrome is unknown, although disturbance of immune mechanisms has been associated with its development. The syndrome may be preceded by respiratory or GI infections or by a surgical procedure, but they do not cause the disorder.

34 Correct answer—A

In Guillain-Barré syndrome, the myelin sheaths of the anterior and posterior spinal roots, ganglia, and spinal and cranial nerves demyelinate and degenerate; this initially causes inflammation and edema and eventually leads to sensory and motor impairment. Loss of pigmented neurons occurs in Parkinson's disease; defective impulse transmission between nerve and muscle cells, in myasthenia gravis; and unexplained loss of basal ganglia cells, in Huntington's disease.

35 Correct answer—A

Guillain-Barré syndrome may lead to loss of the gag and swallowing reflexes, which greatly increases the risk of aspiration. The other choices are not associated with this disorder. When cranial nerves are involved, the seventh cranial (facial) nerve is affected most often, producing bilateral weakness that prevents the patient from wrinkling her forehead or closing her eyes; ptosis and facial twitching do not occur. The patient with Guillain-Barré syndrome typically complains of hyperacusis (abnormal sensitivity to sound), not impaired hearing.

36 Correct answer—D

Although it usually is a slow process, complete recovery is the most likely outcome for a patient with Guillain-Barré syndrome. Exacerbations are uncommon, as is death. Chronic infections are not associated with Guillain-Barré syndrome.

37 Correct answer—A

Transection of the spinal cord at level C5 causes decreased respiratory function because of damage to the nerves that control the heart, respirations, and all vessels and organs below the point of injury. This change in respiratory function is permanent. Loss of respiratory function would indicate damage to the nerves that innervate the diaphragm, which are between levels C1 and C3; such injury usually is rapidly fatal.

38 Correct answer—D

The kinetic therapy (Roto Rest) bed provides slow, continuous side-to-side motion. The air-fluidized (Clinitron) bed uses a flotation system to reduce contact pressure, preventing pressure ulcers; however, it does not provide any motion. The wedge (Stryker) frame allows manual side-to-side rotation to place the patient in a prone or supine position, but it does not provide continuous motion. The circular electric (CircOlectric) bed rotates the patient from head to toe, not from side to side; this type of bed may not be used for a patient with a spinal cord injury because it causes increased spinal movement and compression when rotating the patient vertically.

39 Correct answer—B

Because the patient's spinal cord is transected, he will have no sensory function below the C5 level and cannot experience abdominal pain or tenderness. To assess for intra-abdominal bleeding and stress ulcers, the nurse must rely on objective signs, such as expanding abdominal girth, melena, and a gradual drop in hematocrit.

40 Correct answer—A

Cerebrospinal fluid (CSF) analysis showing increased lymphocytes and oligoclonal immunoglobulin G helps confirm a diagnosis of multiple sclerois (MS). Other helpful diagnostic procedures include CT, nuclear magnetic resonance, and magnetic resonance imaging. Skull X-rays, electroencephalography, and electromyography do not help diagnose MS.

41 Correct answer—A

Areas of demyelination in the main motor pathways (pyramidal tracts) of the spinal cord slow or stop impulse conduction, causing such symptoms as spastic weakness of the lower extremities and bladder and bladder dysfunction. Degeneration of nerve cells in the extrapyramidal system occurs with Parkinson's disease. A sudden, excessive discharge from cerebral neurons results in seizure activity. Dilation of the walls of a cerebral artery is a cerebral aneurysm.

42 Correct answer—B

Involuntary, rhythmic, and rapid jerking of the eyeballs is nystagmus, which may be caused by a central nervous system lesion or by a disturbance in the endolymph fluid. Diplopia is double vision.

Hemianopia is defective vision or blindness in half the visual field of one eye. Esophoria is a tendency of the eye when covered to drift toward the nose.

43 Correct answer—C

After the patient has had a myelogram using a water-soluble contrast medium, the nurse should elevate the head of the bed 15 to 30 degrees to reduce the medium's rate of upward dispersion, preventing such complications as seizures and transient encephalopathy. The nurse should encourage high fluid intake after a myelogram to replace leakage of CSF and to maintain adequate hydration. Monitoring the patient's level of consciousness is not necessary because a myelogram will not alter it. The physician may specify a recumbent position for 12 to 24 hours after the procedure if an oil-based iodine compound is used; this position helps prevent headache and may help reduce CSF leakage.

44 Correct answer—C

Baclofen (Lioresal) should not be discontinued abruptly; this may cause hallucinations. The patient should take this drug with food or milk to prevent GI upset. She should not take baclofen only when symptoms are present; to maintain a therapeutic drug level, she must follow the prescribed dosage schedule (5 mg P.O. three times daily for 3 days, then 10 mg P.O. three times daily increased according to response to a maximum of 20 mg four times daily). Baclofen does not affect urine output.

45 Correct answer—B

If the bladder is overdistended, blood circulation through the bladder slows, lowering its resistance to infection; therefore, the patient should follow the self-catherization schedule to prevent urinary tract infections. Following the schedule will not promote independence, permit more normal sexual relations, or preserve bladder tone.

46 Correct answer—B

Receptive (or sensory) aphasia, the inability to understand written or spoken words, is caused by damage to Wernicke's area of the brain. Damage to Broca's area causes expressive (or motor) aphasia, the inability to speak and write. Brodmann's area is associated with eye movement and pupillary change. The foramen magnum is an anatomic structure of the brain—the opening through which the spinal cord forms a continuous connection with the brain—that is not related to aphasia.

47 Correct answer—A

The long-term goal for the patient should focus on rehabilitating him to promote the highest possible level of physical, mental, and social functioning. Maintaining respiratory function is a priority during the acute phase of a cerebrovascular accident, not a long-term goal; providing respite care services, although important for the caregiver, is not a long-term goal either. Cognitive deficits, which are caused by brain damage, cannot be corrected.

48 Correct answer—C

The ocular pain that accompanies acute closed-angle glaucoma is not caused by increased intracranial pressure but by increased intraocular tension resulting from an imbalance between the formation and reabsorption of aqueous humor. Nausea and vomiting, rainbows or halos around lights, and cloudy, blurred vision are all clinical manifestations of acute closed-angle glaucoma; they are caused by sharply increased intraocular pressure and by ischemia of the ocular nervous system.

49 Correct answer—B

Tonometry testing evaluates intraocular pressure, which normally ranges between 12 and 21 mm Hg; it is used to confirm a diagnosis of acute closed-angle glaucoma or to detect chronic or secondary glaucoma. Another examination, called gonioscopy, may be performed to determine the angle between the iris and the cornea. The patient's ability to focus on close objects is tested with the Snellen chart; refractory errors, such as myopia, presbyopia, and hyperopia, indicate abnormalities in the eye's ability to focus rays on the retina. Direct visualization of the retina requires the use of a slit-lamp biomicroscope with a concave lens. The corneal reflex is tested by lightly touching a wisp of cotton to the cornea, which should cause the eye to blink.

50 Correct answer—D

When administering pilocarpine (Isopto Carpine) eye drops, the nurse must take precautions to prevent the absorption of medication and infectious debris through the lacrimal duct. Tilting the patient's head backward and inclining it slightly to the affected side prevents the absorption of pilocarpine into the systemic circulation. The nurse should not instill the medication in the inner canthus because this would promote absorption of the medication and debris via the lacrimal duct. Moving the eye or squeezing the eyelids tightly would cause the medication to be expelled.

51 Correct answer—C

Pilocarpine induces miosis and spasms of accommodation. The decrease in intraocular pressure occurs when the pupil contracts, widening the angle between the cornea and the iris and promoting the outflow of aqueous humor. Increased lacrimation occurs infrequently. Pilocarpine does not dilate the pupils or increase sensitivity to light.

52 Correct answer—A

Acetazolamide (Diamox), a carbonic anhydrase inhibitor, diminishes the rate of aqueous humor formation in the eye, which decreases intraocular pressure. Because acetazolamide also promotes diuresis by inhibiting carbonic anhydrase activity in the proximal renal tubule, the nurse must monitor the patient's urine output during drug therapy to prevent fluid and electrolyte imbalances. Acetazolamide does not affect pupillary response to light; therefore, the patient should not be sensitive to light. Raising the bed's side rails, which helps prevent injuries, would be necessary only if toxicity developed, lowering the patient's level of consciousness.

53 Correct answer—A

Anticholinergic drugs, such as atropine, produce pupillary dilation, consequently impairing the channels that regulate the outflow of aqueous humor from the eye; this may precipitate an acute attack of glaucoma. Anticholinergic drugs also have an antisecretory action, suppressing lacrimation. Their mydriatic and cycloplegic actions prevent strong contractions by blocking the responses of the iris sphincter muscle and the ciliary muscle of the lens to cholinergic stimulation. Anticholinergic drugs do not cause pupillary contraction.

54 Correct answer—C

The primary purpose of a peripheral iridectomy is to enhance the drainage of aqueous humor from the anterior chamber of the eye. Normally, aqueous fluid flows through the anterior chamber and exits through the canal of Schlemm; acute closed-angle glaucoma blocks or narrows the canal, impairing fluid drainage. Acute closed-angle glaucoma does not commonly result in blood entering the anterior chamber, and a peripheral iridectomy is not performed to prevent this. The procedure does not affect production of vitreous humor, the jellylike substance of the posterior chamber that maintains the shape of the eyeball. The procedure is not done to dilate the pupil; pupillary dilation is a clinical manifestation of acute closed-angle glaucoma and would be present before the procedure.

55 Correct answer—B

The crystalline lens normally is transparent. Physical and chemical changes in the eye may cause opaque spots called cataracts, which cause a slow, painless decrease in visual acuity. Excision is the only repair for a cataract. An abnormal fold of membrane extending from the sclera to the cornea is called a pterygium. Edema of the optic disc, common in individuals with intracranial tumors, is called papilledema. A blind spot in the visual field is called a scotoma; it may be caused by retinal damage following intraocular hemorrhage or inflammation of the choroid.

56 Correct answer—B

The lens is a biconvex crystalline body enclosed in a transparent capsule and suspended by special ligaments; it changes shape to focus light rays properly on the retina. Photosensitive nerve endings in the retina called rods and cones transmit visual impulses to the brain when properly stimulated. The choroid, a highly vascular middle layer of the eyeball, provides nourishment to the eye. The pupil, the circular opening in the center of the iris, dilates and contracts according to light intensity, regulating the amount of light that enters the eye.

57 Correct answer—D

Cyclopentolate (Cyclogyl), commonly administered approximately 2 hours before surgery, dilates the pupil; this dilation facilitates cataract extraction through the pupil. Cyclopentolate does not promote pupil contraction or increase the production of aqueous humor. This drug may increase intraocular pressure, but this is an adverse effect, not its primary purpose.

58 Correct answer—B

Meperidine (Demerol) and hydroxyzine (Vistaril), administered preoperatively, have a sedative effect; raising the bed's side rails ensures the patient's safety when the medications take effect. To promote patient comfort and safety, the nurse should take the patient's vital signs and ensure that she has voided before administering the medications. Checking the patient's pupillary reaction to light would be appropriate if she received morphine but serves no purpose with these medications.

59 Correct answer—A

Some eye pain is not unusual after surgery; however, sudden pain after cataract extraction may indicate increased intraocular pressure and hemorrhage, which must be treated promptly. Swelling of the eyelids is expected after surgery and should subside within a few days. Hazy vision is fairly common, especially if an ophthalmic ointment has been applied; it does not indicate an immediate danger. Slight nausea is common as well; the nurse does not have to report this to the physician immediately unless the patient develops severe retching and vomiting, which may increase intraocular pressure.

60 Correct answer—D

After cataract extraction, the patient must wear an eye patch. After this eye patch is removed, the patient may not have to wear another one during the day; however, she must wear an eye shield while sleeping to prevent accidental trauma to the eye. Deep breathing is beneficial, but coughing is contraindicated because it may increase intraocular pressure. A low-fiber diet is contraindicated because it may lead to constipation and straining during bowel movements, which increases intraocular pressure. The patient should avoid eye muscle exercises and any other unnecessary eye movement, which may interfere with healing.

61 Correct answer—C

Pulling the pinna up and back permits better visualization of an adult's external auditory canal. Pulling the pinna down and back permits better visualization with a child. Depressing the tragus, the triangular cartilaginous projection over the external opening of the ear canal, would obstruct visualization. Holding the otoscope upside-down in the dominant hand is a personal preference that would not affect visualization.

62 Correct answer—A

To perform the Rinne test, the nurse holds the base of an activated tuning fork on the mastoid bone until the patient can no longer hear the vibrations, then holds the still-vibrating fork near the external ear; a negative result means the patient hears vibrations longer or louder by bone conduction than by air conduction, which indicates a conductive hearing loss. A person without a hearing problem should hear the sound about twice as long by air conduction. Sound heard poorly by both air and bone conduction may indicate sensorineural hearing loss.

CHAPTER 4

Gastrointestinal System

Questions

1 During physical assessment of a patient's abdomen, the nurse should perform the four basic techniques in the following order:

A. Auscultation, palpation, inspection, percussion
B. Inspection, auscultation, percussion, palpation
C. Inspection, auscultation, palpation, percussion
D. Percussion, auscultation, palpation, inspection

2 Mr. F. is scheduled for an upper GI series. Which intervention should the nurse perform after the procedure?

A. Testing stool for occult blood
B. Auscultating the abdomen for bowel sounds
C. Assessing for the gag reflex
D. Forcing fluids

3 Mr. K., a patient with a duodenal ulcer, is placed on a bland diet and receives medications to decrease gastric acidity. Which medication reduces hydrochloric acid secretion?

A. Cimetidine (Tagamet)
B. Aluminum hydroxide (Amphojel)
C. Sucralfate (Carafate)
D. Aspirin

4 Mr. K.'s ulcer perforates the peritoneal cavity. To relieve the pain caused by perforation, Mr. K. is likely to:

A. Lie on his left side
B. Turn onto his stomach
C. Rigidly maintain the supine position
D. Draw his knees up to his abdomen

5 A patient who has undergone a Billroth II operation may prevent dumping syndrome by:

A. Drinking water with meals
B. Remaining upright after meals
C. Avoiding bending over
D. Lying down after meals

6 Which statement accurately describes a LeVeen shunt?

A. It is a tube with a one-way valve placed between the peritoneal cavity and the vena cava
B. It shunts blood around the liver to the vena cava
C. It removes ascitic fluid when used with a syringe
D. It replaces ascitic fluid with protein-enriched fluid

7 Mortality after a liver transplant has improved markedly since 1980. All of the following patients now are considered candidates for a liver transplant *except:*

A. Those with irreversible, otherwise untreatable hepatic disease
B. Those with cirrhosis from chronic hepatitis B infection
C. Those with a history of multiple intra-abdominal surgical procedures
D. Those with alcoholic cirrhosis

8 When administering hepatitis B vaccine, the nurse should:

A. Inject it in the deltoid muscle
B. Inject it in the gluteal muscle
C. Use a ½″ needle
D. Change the needle after withdrawing the vaccine

9 The main pathogenic agent involved in hepatic failure is:

A. Lipase
B. Ammonia
C. Potassium
D. Albumin

10 The characteristic symptom of impending hepatic coma is:

A. Ataxia
B. Asterixis
C. Dyskinesia
D. Opisthotonos

11 Which complication may occur in a patient receiving prolonged nasogastric tube feedings?

A. A gastric ulcer resulting from a plugged tube, which prolongs contact between hyperosmotic material and gastric mucosa
B. Trauma to the gastric mucosa caused by the distal end of the tube hardening over time
C. Dislocation of the tube into the esophagus, causing fistulas and diverticula formation
D. Formation of a tracheoesophageal fistula, resulting from breakdown of the posterior esophageal wall

12 Which patient situation might warrant total parenteral nutrition (TPN) therapy?

A. Nonfunctional GI tract and NPO status for more than 5 days
B. Short-term nutritional support to supplement intermittent oral feeding
C. Ability to tolerate administration of up to 3 liters of fluid daily on a short-term basis
D. Long-term enteral therapy after resection of the GI tract above the stomach

13 Many factors contribute to poor nutrition. Which factor is considered the most critical?

A. Ignorance
B. Laziness
C. Faddism
D. Income

14 Assessment of a patient with staphylococcal food poisoning most likely would reveal:

A. Temperature of 102° F (38.9° C), abdominal cramps, chills, and intermittent diarrhea
B. Abdominal cramps, diaphoresis, and chills (no fever)
C. Subnormal temperature (97° F [36.1° C]), continuous diarrhea, and chills
D. Chills, abdominal pain, and bloody diarrhea

SITUATION

Mrs. J., age 65, is admitted to the emergency department complaining of severe lower abdominal pain. The physician suspects diverticular disease and peritonitis.

Questions 15 and 16 refer to this situation.

15 Which assessment finding for Mrs. J. indicates peritonitis?

A. Temperature above 102° F (38.9° C)
B. Diarrhea
C. Shallow respirations
D. Hyperactive bowel sounds

16 Mrs. J. progresses quickly after an exploratory laparotomy. Upon discharge, the nurse instructs Mrs. J. to take all of the following measures *except:*

A. Avoiding constipation
B. Reducing weight if obese
C. Performing activities that increase intra-abdominal pressure
D. Drinking at least eight glasses of water daily

SITUATION

Ms. S., a 35-year-old legal clerk, is admitted to the unit with an acute episode of ulcerative colitis.

Questions 17 to 20 refer to this situation.

17 Which fluid could the nurse give Ms. S. to improve hydration?

A. Orange juice
B. Hot chocolate
C. Weak, warm tea
D. Cola

18 The nurse should perform all of the following interventions for Ms. S. *except:*

A. Providing bed rest
B. Relieving pain
C. Recording fluid intake and output
D. Providing a high-residue, low-protein diet

19 Ms. S.'s condition deteriorates, and the physician schedules a hemicolectomy and ileostomy. Which statement about ileostomies is true?

A. The patient must wear an ostomy appliance at all times
B. The patient must learn to irrigate the canal on a regular basis
C. The patient's stool eventually will be solid
D. The patient likely will experience malabsorption syndrome

20 Before discharge, the nurse should discuss all of the following topics with Ms. S. *except:*

A. The need for an appropriate solvent when removing the appliance
B. The importance of maintaining a low-fiber diet
C. The benefits of immediate vigorous exercise
D. The need to increase fluid intake when perspiring heavily

SITUATION

Mrs. K., an active 62-year-old woman, complains to her physician about difficulty passing stool, mucus in her stools, and a feeling that her bowel is not completely emptied after defecation. Her physician suspects cancer of the descending colon and admits Mrs. K. to the hospital for diagnostic testing. Blood studies reveal a hemoglobin (Hgb) level of 14 g/dl and a hematocrit (HCT) level of 42%.

Questions 21 to 24 refer to this situation.

21 After testing confirms the diagnosis of cancer of the descending colon, the physician schedules Mrs. K. for an abdominoperineal resection with a permanent colostomy. Which procedure is *not* indicated in preparing this patient for surgery?

A. Maintaining a low-residue or liquid diet to decrease the amount of fecal waste in the bowel
B. Administering antibiotics for several days before surgery to sterilize the bowel
C. Administering enemas to empty the bowel
D. Transfusing two units of whole blood to raise Hgb and HCT levels to normal

22 When giving Mrs. K. instructions for irrigating her colostomy at home, the nurse tells her to call her physician if:

A. The stoma's color changes from pink to black
B. She experiences abdominal cramping during irrigation
C. She encounters resistance when inserting the catheter
D. The irrigating solution backflows

23 The nurse recognizes that Mrs. K.'s husband is anxious and having difficulty accepting his wife's physical changes. Which nursing action would be most helpful to Mr. K.?

A. Communicate to Mr. K. that his feelings are only temporary and will go away
B. Explain to Mr. K. that there is no reason why he and his wife cannot have normal sexual relations
C. Encourage Mr. K. to attend his wife's patient-teaching sessions and to participate in her care
D. Ignore Mr. K.'s feelings; the nurse's priority is the patient

24 Which postdischarge behavior would indicate that Mrs. K. does *not* understand her diet?

A. Avoiding gas-forming foods
B. Avoiding bulk-forming foods
C. Eating slowly
D. Avoiding carbonated beverages

SITUATION

Mr. G., age 60, is admitted to the hospital with ascites and jaundice to rule out cirrhosis of the liver.

Questions 25 to 29 refer to this situation.

25 Which laboratory test result indicates cirrhosis?

A. Decreased red blood cell count
B. Decreased serum acid phosphatase level
C. Elevated white blood cell count
D. Elevated serum alanine aminotransferase (formerly serum glutamic-pyruvic transaminase) level

26 The physician schedules Mr. G. for a liver biopsy to confirm the diagnosis of cirrhosis. Which crucial information should the nurse tell Mr. G. before the procedure?

A. He should hold his breath on exhalation when the biopsy needle is inserted
B. The procedure is painless
C. He must maintain a side-lying position after the procedure
D. Pressure will be applied to his right side after the procedure

27 The biopsy confirms the diagnosis of cirrhosis. Mr. G. is at increased risk for excessive bleeding primarily because of:

A. Impaired clotting mechanisms
B. Varix formation
C. Inadequate nutrition
D. Trauma from invasive procedures

28 Mr. G. develops hepatic encephalopathy. Which clinical manifestations are most common with this condition?

A. Increased urine output
B. Decreased tendon reflexes
C. Altered attention span
D. Hypotension

29 Once Mr. G. has regained consciousness, the physician orders 50 ml of lactulose (Chronulac) P.O. every 2 hours. Later in the day, Mr. G. complains of diarrhea. The nurse's best response would be:

A. "I'll see if your physician is in the hospital"
B. "Maybe you're reacting to the drug; I'll withhold the next dose"
C. "I'll lower the dosage as ordered so the drug causes two to four stools daily"
D. "Frequent bowel movements are needed to reduce sodium levels"

SITUATION

Mr. B., a 27-year-old construction worker, is returned to the unit after surgical repair of an inguinal hernia (herniorrhaphy).

Questions 30 and 31 refer to this situation.

30 Mr. B. reports scrotal soreness and swelling. The nurse's first action should be:

A. Applying an ice bag to the scrotum
B. Giving him pain medication as ordered
C. Encouraging him to stand up and walk slowly for a short time
D. Increasing his fluid intake

31 Before Mr. B.'s discharge, the nurse lists certain activity restrictions for him. Which restriction is *not* necessary for this patient?

A. No driving for 2 to 4 weeks
B. No heavy lifting, pushing, or pulling for 6 weeks
C. No sexual activity for at least 3 weeks
D. No walking for 2 weeks

SITUATION

Mrs. L., age 67, is admitted to the hospital with a hiatal hernia. She complains of symptoms associated with esophageal reflux.

Questions 32 and 33 refer to this situation.

32 To minimize Mrs. L.'s discomfort, the nurse should recommend that she take all of the following measures *except:*

A. Avoiding constipation
B. Sleeping with her head elevated
C. Wearing a girdle to keep her stomach pulled upward
D. Avoiding tomatoes and greasy food

33 The physician prescribes magaldrate (Riopan) for Mrs. L. to relieve her discomfort. This antacid's adverse effects include:

A. Constipation or diarrhea
B. Restlessness and insomnia
C. Urinary urgency and increased salivation
D. Abdominal distention and excess flatus

SITUATION

Mr. N., a 42-year-old accountant, is admitted to the hospital with intestinal obstruction. A flat-plate X-ray of the abdomen shows a mass, which may be malignant.

Questions 34 and 35 refer to this situation.

34 Preliminary assessment findings for Mr. N. probably will include:

A. A flat abdomen with bowel sounds audible in all quadrants
B. Tachycardia and hypertension
C. Vomiting, constipation, and abdominal distention
D. Flushed skin and diaphoresis

35 Which type of tube will Mr. N.'s physician require for intestinal decompression?

A. Miller-Abbott
B. Levin
C. Salem sump
D. Ewald

SITUATION

Mrs. G., a 45-year-old Native American, is admitted to a hospital with severe abdominal pain in the right upper quadrant, flatulence, and indigestion. The physician suspects gallbladder disease.

Question 36 refers to this situation.

36 Which assessment finding does *not* indicate a high risk of developing gallbladder disease?

A. Race
B. Active life-style
C. Obesity
D. Estrogen therapy

Diagnostic testing confirms a diagnosis of active cholelithiasis (gallstones); the physician schedules Mrs. G. for a cholecystectomy and exploration of the common bile duct.

Questions 37 and 38 continue the situation.

37 The evening before surgery, Mrs. G. complains of intense pruritus. This condition most likely is caused by:

A. An allergy to her gallstones
B. Anxiety about her impending surgery
C. Biliary colic
D. Deposition of bile salts in the peripheral circulation

38 Mrs. G's physician schedules a cholangiogram before removal of her T tube. Mrs. G. asks about the purpose of this procedure. Which response should the nurse give?

A. "It determines whether all of the stones have been removed"
B. "It shows whether the remaining stones are calcified"
C. "It identifies spasms of the sphincter of Oddi"
D. "It provides access to any remaining stones"

SITUATION

Mrs. D., a 40-year-old banker, is admitted to the medical unit with a tentative diagnosis of hepatitis A.

Questions 39 to 42 refer to this situation.

39 Which laboratory test result is most conclusive is confirming a diagnosis of hepatitis A?

A. An elevated serum alanine aminotransferase level
B. Acholic stool
C. Hepatitis A virus antibodies (anti-HAV IgM) in serum
D. An elevated serum alkaline phosphatase level

40 The physician determines that Mrs. D. is in the icteric stage of hepatitis A infection. Which nursing intervention is *not* appropriate during this stage?

A. Forcing fluids (3,000 ml or more daily)
B. Administering vitamin K as ordered
C. Encouraging ambulation to prevent pneumonia
D. Providing mittens for the patient

41 Which discharge instruction should the nurse stress with Mrs. D.?

A. "Wear a medical alert bracelet at all times"
B. "Never donate blood"
C. "Use a condom during sexual intercourse"
D. "Wash your hands before and after bowel movements"

42 Mrs. D.'s husband was exposed to hepatitis A. Which treatment should the nurse expect the physician to order for Mr. D.?

A. Immune serum globulin
B. Vaccine containing hepatitis B surface antigen
C. Bacille Calmette-Guérin vaccine
D. Tetanus toxoid

SITUATION

Mr. J., a 50-year-old postal worker, is admitted to the hospital with acute pancreatitis.

Questions 43 to 49 refer to this situation.

43 If Mr. J. begins to exhibit muscle twitching and irritability, the nurse should:

A. Administer an analgesic because the symptoms are probably caused by the pain
B. Call the physician because the patient may have hypocalcemia
C. Reassure the patient that this is common among people who abuse alcohol
D. Check his serum amylase level

44 Which position might Mr. J. assume during episodes of acute pancreatitis?

A. Knees flexed toward abdomen
B. Supine with legs extended
C. Trendelenburg's position
D. Lithotomy position

45 The physician orders blood glucose measurements for Mr. J. every 4 hours. During the acute stage of pancreatitis, the patient typically is:

A. Hypoglycemic
B. Hyperglycemic
C. Normoglycemic
D. Uremic

46 The physician orders an analgesic for Mr. J.'s pancreatitis pain. Which drug is preferred for pain relief?

A. Morphine
B. Codeine
C. Acetaminophen with codeine (Tylenol #3)
D. Meperidine (Demerol)

47 The nurse should expect Mr. J.'s meals to be:

A. High-fat, low-carbohydrate
B. Low-protein, low-carbohydrate
C. High-carbohydrate, low-fat
D. Large and high-caloric

48 Which foods would be most appropriate for Mr. J. while he recovers from pancreatitis?

A. Eggs, milk, and cheese
B. Coffee, tea, and cola
C. Bread, gelatin, and cereal
D. Pork, bacon, and cheeseburgers

49 The nurse's discharge planning for Mr. J. includes dietary teaching. Which instruction would *not* be appropriate for Mr. J.?

A. "Avoid coffee"
B. "Avoid spicy food"
C. "Avoid large meals"
D. "Avoid antacids"

SITUATION

Ms. G., age 26, comes to the medical clinic to speak with the nurse. Ms. G. is 5-ft., 1-in. tall and weighs 280 lb. She tells the nurse she is having difficulty walking and wants to lose weight.

Questions 50 to 52 refer to this situation.

50 Weight loss is best accomplished through behavior modification. When establishing Ms. G.'s program, the nurse might begin by:

A. Allowing her to set the rules
B. Acting as a "warden" on her eating habits
C. Planning a strict schedule for her to follow
D. Granting privileges for accomplishments

51 Which nursing history finding probably will relate significantly to Ms. G.'s obesity?

A. Leisure time and social activities
B. Birth weight and length
C. Previous illnesses
D. Parents' and siblings' height and weight

52 Several weeks after starting a diet, Ms. G. mentions that she is taking various measures to adjust her eating habits. Which measure would *not* be appropriate?

A. Eating slowly during meals
B. Decreasing the portions of food eaten
C. Keeping no snack food in the house
D. Skipping breakfast every day

SITUATION

Mr. J., age 59, was admitted to the hospital with chronic gastroenteritis. To meet Mr. J.'s nutritional needs, the physician orders total parenteral nutrition (TPN) via a central venous catheter.

Questions 53 to 56 refer to this situation.

53 To prevent air embolus formation while inserting Mr. J.'s TPN catheter, the nurse should instruct him to:

A. Pant
B. Use ballottement
C. Perform Valsalva's maneuver
D. Perform an isometric maneuver

54 Which measure should the nurse take to ensure adequate assessment and prevent infection while Mr. J. is on TPN?

A. Changing TPN tubing as needed
B. Administering no medications or blood products through the TPN line
C. Changing TPN dressing once a week
D. Taking vital signs every 12 hours

55 Which finding indicates dislodgement of Mr. J.'s central venous catheter?

A. Rebound hypoglycemia
B. Profuse diuresis
C. Muscle spasms
D. Shoulder pain and facial edema

56 Which guideline should the nurse remember when choosing food for Mr. J.'s menu when he is taken off TPN therapy?

A. Foods selected should be chemically and mechanically nonirritating and high in calories, protein, and minerals
B. Keeping in mind the patient's likes and dislikes, foods selected should be high in residue and fat to stimulate motility
C. Low-protein foods should be introduced slowly to reduce damage to the renal membrane
D. Certain fluids, such as cocoa and carbonated drinks, tend to increase upper jejunal digestion and reduce folate deficiency

---

SITUATION

Mr. M., a 66-year-old patient admitted to the hospital with a cerebrovascular accident, receives nasogastric tube feedings for nutritional support.

Questions 57 to 59 refer to this situation.

57 Which intervention should the nurse implement in case Mr. M. aspirates his tube feedings?

A. Aspirating residue every 8 hours
B. Reinstilling all residual feedings regardless of color or consistency
C. Allowing the patient to lie on his left side to delay gastric emptying and to allow full digestion
D. Having suction available at all times, especially if the patient has an impaired gag reflex

58 Which assessment measure should the nurse carry out to protect Mr. M. from a potential fluid volume deficit?

A. Assessing for dehydration, which may be caused by diarrhea, excessive protein intake, or osmotic diuresis
B. Observing for osmotic diuresis, which may result from a high glucose load when the infusion rate is decreased
C. Assessing for lethargy, disorientation, and engorged neck veins
D. Observing for constipation and abdominal cramping

59 Before Mr. M.'s discharge, the nurse meets with him to plan his management of tube feedings at home. Which instruction should the nurse emphasize?

A. "The formula should be at room temperature by the time administration ends"
B. "Irrigations of 25 to 50 ml of sterile water every 24 hours ensures tube patency"
C. "Position during the feedings is determined by comfort, not by any other factors or complications"
D. "Observe for signs of electrolyte imbalance or bacterial infection to prevent further complications"

Answer sheet

	A B C D		A B C D
1	○ ○ ○ ○	31	○ ○ ○ ○
2	○ ○ ○ ○	32	○ ○ ○ ○
3	○ ○ ○ ○	33	○ ○ ○ ○
4	○ ○ ○ ○	34	○ ○ ○ ○
5	○ ○ ○ ○	35	○ ○ ○ ○
6	○ ○ ○ ○	36	○ ○ ○ ○
7	○ ○ ○ ○	37	○ ○ ○ ○
8	○ ○ ○ ○	38	○ ○ ○ ○
9	○ ○ ○ ○	39	○ ○ ○ ○
10	○ ○ ○ ○	40	○ ○ ○ ○
11	○ ○ ○ ○	41	○ ○ ○ ○
12	○ ○ ○ ○	42	○ ○ ○ ○
13	○ ○ ○ ○	43	○ ○ ○ ○
14	○ ○ ○ ○	44	○ ○ ○ ○
15	○ ○ ○ ○	45	○ ○ ○ ○
16	○ ○ ○ ○	46	○ ○ ○ ○
17	○ ○ ○ ○	47	○ ○ ○ ○
18	○ ○ ○ ○	48	○ ○ ○ ○
19	○ ○ ○ ○	49	○ ○ ○ ○
20	○ ○ ○ ○	50	○ ○ ○ ○
21	○ ○ ○ ○	51	○ ○ ○ ○
22	○ ○ ○ ○	52	○ ○ ○ ○
23	○ ○ ○ ○	53	○ ○ ○ ○
24	○ ○ ○ ○	54	○ ○ ○ ○
25	○ ○ ○ ○	55	○ ○ ○ ○
26	○ ○ ○ ○	56	○ ○ ○ ○
27	○ ○ ○ ○	57	○ ○ ○ ○
28	○ ○ ○ ○	58	○ ○ ○ ○
29	○ ○ ○ ○	59	○ ○ ○ ○
30	○ ○ ○ ○		

Answers and rationales

1 Correct answer—B

Physical assessment of the abdomen consists of inspection, auscultation, percussion, and palpation. Visual inspection is always the first step in any physical assessment. Although auscultation is performed last during physical assessment of other body systems, the nurse must use this technique before percussion and palpation of the abdomen because they may alter intestinal activity and bowel sounds. Palpation of the abdomen should be performed after percussion because it may cause pain or disturb fluid, masses, and the position of organs, interfering with any assessment techniques performed afterward.

2 Correct answer—D

For an upper GI series, the patient ingests barium as a contrast medium; because remaining barium could harden and cause intestinal blockage, the nurse should force fluids to aid evacuation. The patient may receive a laxative also, according to institutional protocol. The stool will be minimal and contain barium. Testing for occult blood and auscultating the abdomen for bowel sounds would not help eliminate barium from the patient's body, which is the goal of nursing intervention after an upper GI series. Assessing for the gag reflex is unnecessary; the procedure does not affect this reflex.

3 Correct answer—A

Cimetidine (Tagamet), a histamine$_2$-receptor antagonist, decreases hydrochloric acid secretion, facilitating ulcer healing. Antacids, such as aluminum hydroxide (Amphojel), provide symptomatic relief from ulcer pain by neutralizing gastric acid. Sucralfate (Carafate), an agent used to treat duodenal ulcers, coats the ulcer site with a protective barrier resistant to acid. Aspirin, which is associated with ulcer development, is contraindicated in the patient with a duodenal ulcer.

4 Correct answer—D

Characteristically, the patient will draw his knees up to his abdomen or bend over, which relieves the pain by decreasing the tension on the abdominal muscles. The patient may turn on his left or right side or turn onto his stomach, but these positions will not relieve the pain. The patient may assume the supine position, but he is likely to move about in efforts to become more comfortable, not remain rigid.

5 Correct answer—**D**

Lying down after meals helps prevent dumping syndrome. The Billroth II operation—removal of part of the stomach and duodenum and anastomosis of the resected stomach to the jejunum—causes rapid gastric emptying. A concentrated mass of chyme rapidly entering the small intestines results in fluid being drawn into the bowel, decreasing vascular fluid; this decrease leads to dizziness, sweating, palpitations, and other signs and symptoms of dumping syndrome. Lying down after eating slows peristalsis and allows increased breakdown of food by gastric juices, preventing the sudden emptying of chyme into the intestines and the resulting dumping syndrome. Drinking water or other fluids with meals and remaining upright after eating are contraindicated because these actions accelerate gastric emptying. The patient need not avoid bending over, which does not affect gastric emptying.

6 Correct answer—**A**

The LeVeen shunt is a tube placed subcutaneously between the peritoneal cavity and superior vena cava; its pressure-activated, one-way valve allows peritoneal fluid to enter the vascular space but prevents backflow of blood into the tube. Shunting of blood around the liver (portacaval shunt) is a surgical procedure, not a device. A paracentesis aspirates ascitic fluid with a needle or trocar connected to a syringe or vacuum bottle. An albumin or plasma infusion replaces protein.

7 Correct answer—**C**

Although improved surgical technique and preparation has increased the number of liver transplant candidates, patients who have had multiple intra-abdominal surgical procedures are not considered candidates because those previous procedures increase blood loss during liver transplant, complicate surgery because of adhesions, and increase early mortality. Those with irreversible liver disease, such as fulminating liver failure and biliary cirrhosis, are candidates for liver transplant. Although the practice is somewhat controversial, transplants may be given to patients with cirrhosis from chronic hepatitis B infection; however, it is necessary to eliminate the infection before surgery and prevent its recurrence afterward. Patients with alcoholic cirrhosis also are candidates if they have demonstrated complete recovery from alcoholism.

8 Correct answer—A

When administering hepatitis B vaccine, the nurse should inject it in the deltoid muscle instead of the gluteal muscle, which absorbs the vaccine erratically. The nurse should use a 1½ ″ needle for all I.M. injections. Because the vaccine does not damage subcutaneous tissue, the nurse does not need to change the needle after withdrawing the vaccine.

9 Correct answer—B

Intestinal digestion is a major source of ammonia; this ammonia is converted to urea in the liver and is then excreted by the kidneys. When the liver cannot convert ammonia to urea, large amounts of ammonia enter the systemic circulation and produce toxic neurologic effects. The other choices are not involved with hepatic failure.

10 Correct answer—B

Asterixis, or flapping tremors, may involve the arms and legs; when a patient with impending hepatic coma holds his arms and hands stretched out, a series of rapid flexion and extension movements of the hands occur. These tremors are caused by the accumulation of ammonia and other toxic metabolites in the blood. Ataxia refers to lack of muscle coordination usually seen with lesions of the sensory pathways or cerebellum as well as with sedative or antiseizure drug toxicity. Dyskinesia refers to impairment of the power of voluntary movements, resulting in fragmented or incomplete movements; it may also manifest itself as an idiosyncratic reaction to psychotropic drugs. Opisthotonos, extreme arching of the back with retraction of the head, occurs during the tonic phase of a generalized tonic-clonic seizure.

11 Correct answer—B

Positioning the tube against the stomach mucosa may result in trauma because the distal end of the tube hardens over time. Plugging of the tube may occur with nasogastric (NG) feedings; however, ulcerations would occur in the nares rather than the gastric area. Dislocation of the tube into the esophagus would cause aspiration of all material, not the formation of fistulas and diverticula. Tracheoesophageal fistulas may form if a breakdown of the anterior, not posterior, wall of the esophagus occurs because of prolonged contact between the NG tube and a tracheostomy tube.

12 Correct answer—A

When a patient has a nonfunctioning GI tract and requires rest from the processes of ingestion, digestion, and absorption for more than 5 days, total parenteral nutrition (TPN) is warranted. Short-term nutritional support for a patient who can tolerate oral feedings intermittently calls for tube feedings. Partial parenteral nutrition may be used for short-term nutritional therapy, but not long-term therapy. The ability to tolerate the administration of 3 liters of fluid daily is not a condition or requirement for TPN; fluids are given at a rate the patient can tolerate (usually less than 0.25 liter/hour), and their compositions are altered to meet the patient's nutritional needs. Obstructions of the GI tract above the stomach requiring long-term enteral therapy necessitate gastrostomy or jejunostomy tube insertion, not TPN.

13 Correct answer—D

Although ignorance, laziness, and food fads may contribute to a patient's poor nutrition, income is the most critical factor in why people select what they eat. Low income affects the ability to purchase a sufficient quantity of necessary foods.

14 Correct answer—B

Clinical manifestations of staphylococcal food poisoning include abdominal cramps, diaphoresis, and chills, with no fever; these signs and symptoms are caused by enterotoxins that impair intestinal absorption and produce acute gastroenteritis with an incubation period of 1 to 6 hours. Staphylococcal food poisoning does not cause fever (like salmonella food poisoning does) or subnormal body temperatures. Although diarrhea may last for 8 to 24 hours, it is not intermittent or bloody. This condition, although acute, resolves spontaneously; treatment is symptomatic.

15 Correct answer—C

The patient with peritonitis typically breathes shallowly because movement increases abdominal pain. Peritonitis may increase the patient's temperature, but fever is usually low-grade (below 101° F [38.3° C]). The patient may experience constipation, not diarrhea. Bowel sounds are absent, not hyperactive, with peritonitis.

16 Correct answer—C

The patient should avoid activities that increase intra-abdominal pressure, such as bending and lifting; increased intra-abdominal pressure may tear sutures and exacerbate diverticula. Avoiding constipation will decrease episodes of diverticulitis, as will reducing weight. A high fluid intake helps prevent constipation.

17 Correct answer—C

Weak, warm tea is the least irritating of the beverages listed. Orange juice, hot chocolate, and such carbonated drinks as cola are contraindicated because they may be chemically or mechanically irritating to the bowel.

18 Correct answer—D

Instead of a high-residue, low-protein diet, the nurse should provide low-residue, high-protein meals with vitamin and mineral supplements to meet the patient's nutritional needs. Low residue decreases the amount of fecal waste, allowing the bowel to rest; protein is necessary for tissue regeneration and healing. Bed rest decreases intestinal motility. Relieving pain is a vital intervention because it enhances patient compliance with treatment. Fluid replacement is necessary to maintain homeostasis; therefore, the nurse must record intake and output to guide the procedure.

19 Correct answer—A

Because the bowel drainage is liquid, the patient must wear an ostomy appliance (collection pouch) at all times. Irrigation may be used for colostomy cleaning or regulation, but it is not necessary with an ileostomy. The patient's stool will never be solid because of enzymatic action and the lack of water absorption in the small intestines. Malabsorption is not common after an ileostomy because most of the small intestine, where nutrient absorption occurs, is intact after the procedure.

20 Correct answer—C

After ileostomy surgery, the patient should not exercise vigorously until she is fully healed. The use of a solvent when removing the appliance is important; attempts to pull off the appliance without dissolving the cement will cause severe skin trauma. Although the bowel drainage is watery, the patient should maintain a low-fiber diet to decrease the amount of fecal waste, reducing the risk of bowel irritation. Because fluid and electrolytes, particularly sodium, are lost through perspiration, the patient must replace them by increasing her fluid intake.

21 Correct answer—D

Preoperative transfusion of whole blood is not indicated because the patient's hemoglobin and hematocrit levels are within normal limits. Preparation for any patient undergoing bowel surgery includes a low-residue or liquid diet, antibiotic administration, and enema administration.

22 Correct answer—A

The color of the stoma indicates the adequacy of its blood supply. Darkening from pink to black means the stoma's blood supply has become inadequate, which may lead to necrosis and a nonfunctioning colostomy. This is a medical emergency that the patient must report to her physician immediately. Less serious problems, such as abdominal cramping during irrigation, resistance during catheter insertion, and backflow of the irrigating solution, are common among patients with a colostomy; therefore, discharge instructions include simple techniques to use if these problems occur.

23 Correct answer—C

By encouraging Mr. K. to attend his wife's patient-teaching sessions and to participate in her care, the nurse may alleviate his anxiety and difficulty accepting his wife's physical changes, which is probably related to lack of knowledge and fear of the unknown. The partner of a patient with a colostomy commonly has negative feelings about the patient's body changes. The nurse cannot assume these feelings are temporary or related to the resumption of normal sexual relations. The nurse cannot ignore Mr. K.'s feelings because they will affect Mrs. K.'s acceptance of her colostomy.

24 Correct answer—B

The patient should eat roughage, fresh fruits and vegetables, and other bulk-forming foods to prevent constipation. The patient should avoid gas-forming foods, such as beans and cabbage; eat slowly to avoid swallowing air; and avoid carbonated beverages. These measures will help the patient avoid embarrassment caused by gas in social situations, which commonly leads to withdrawal in patients with a colostomy.

25 Correct answer—D

Alanine aminotransferase, a liver enzyme, is released when liver tissue is damaged; an elevated serum level indicates cirrhosis, although further testing is needed to confirm the diagnosis. The decrease in red blood cells (RBCs) usually is a result of blood loss; although the liver plays a role in RBC formation, this decrease is not diagnostically significant. Increased serum acid phosphatase levels indicate surgical trauma or prostatic cancer; an increase in white blood cells indicates infection.

26 Correct answer—A

To prevent puncture of the diaphragm, the nurse should tell the patient to hold his breath on exhalation when the needle is inserted. Because the patient may feel discomfort during needle insertion, he should not be told the procedure is painless. After the procedure, the patient must lie on his right side on a pillow or sandbag to arrest bleeding; however, this information is not crucial for the patient to know before the procedure.

27 Correct answer—A

Cirrhosis causes decreased absorption of vitamin K; this decrease results in thrombocytopenia, leading to impaired clotting. Although varix formation, inadequate nutrition, and trauma also increase the risk of excessive bleeding, impaired clotting is the most significant factor.

28 Correct answer—C

Hepatic encephalopathy commonly causes altered attention span, as well as tremors, changes in affect, irritability, and lack of coordination followed by disorientation to time, then to place. Ascites, which accompanies hepatic encephalopathy, causes a decrease in intravascular volume, stimulating the release of renin and aldosterone; these hormones cause the kidneys to retain sodium and water, which decreases urine output. Tendon reflexes usually are increased with hepatic encephalopathy until the patient loses consciousness; hypotension rarely occurs with this condition.

29 Correct answer—C

The initial dosage for lactulose (Chronulac) is 50 ml P.O. every 2 hours until diarrhea occurs; the dosage then is lowered as ordered until the drug causes two to four stools daily. Lactulose is prescribed to decrease nitrogenous substrate and reduce toxins in the GI tract and to reduce blood ammonia levels. The nurse does not need to find the patient's physician or withhold the next dose because the drug is having the desired effect. Lactulose is not given to rid the body of such nontoxic substances as sodium.

30 Correct answer—A

The nurse should first apply an ice bag to the scrotum to immediately reduce pain and swelling, which is caused by edema of the tissues surrounding the scrotal cord. Giving medication to reduce the patient's pain would be the next nursing action. The nurse should not encourage the patient to walk without scrotal support if the scrotum is edematous; this would increase the pain and possibly tear the sutures. Increasing the patient's fluid intake would not relieve the pain or swelling.

31 Correct answer—D

The patient does not need to completely avoid walking after discharge. After a herniorrhaphy, the patient must avoid activities that may cause increased intra-abdominal pressure, which may tear sutures or cause hernia recurrence. Moderate walking while performing activities of daily living will not cause increased pressure; however, the patient should not walk for long distances or at a fast pace. Driving, lifting, pushing, pulling, and sexual activity are restricted for certain periods.

32 Correct answer—C

To reduce the symptoms associated with esophageal reflux, the patient should avoid activities that move gastric secretions upward toward the esophageal mucosa; because a girdle's constricting effect moves secretions upward, the patient should not wear one. The patient should take measures to avoid constipation, which results in increased intra-abdominal pressure when the patient attempts to evacuate. Sleeping with the head elevated facilitates gastric emptying, decreasing reflux. The patient should avoid acidic foods, such as tomatoes, as well as greasy foods because they increase reflux.

33 Correct answer—A

The adverse effects of magaldrate (Riopan) include mild constipation or diarrhea, fatigue or weakness, and weight loss. The drug does not cause restlessness, insomnia, urinary urgency, increased salivation, abdominal distention, or excess flatus.

34 Correct answer—C

The patient with an intestinal obstruction will likely experience vomiting, constipation, and abdominal distention. Bowel sounds may not be audible in all quadrants, depending on the location of the obstruction. Tachycardia is likely, but the patient probably will be hypotensive because of dehydration (common in the early acute stage of this condition) or peritonitis. Flushed skin and diaphoresis, which indicate fever, are common only if peritonitis is also present.

35 Correct answer—A

The physician will use the Miller-Abbott tube, a double-lumen tube with an inflatable balloon, to decompress the patient's intestine. The Levin tube is a single-lumen nasogastric tube used to decompress the stomach. The Salem sump tube is a double-lumen tube used for stomach decompression. The Ewald tube is a large-bore tube used to evacuate the stomach.

36 Correct answer—B

A sedentary life-style, not an active one, indicates a high risk of gallbladder disease. The patient's race affects the risk of gallbladder disease; recent studies show a high incidence of cholelithiasis (gallstones) among Native American women over age 30, and gallbladder disease is more common among Whites than among Asians and Blacks. Obesity, postmenopausal estrogen therapy, use of oral contraceptives, a family history of gallbladder disease, and multiparity are also high-risk factors. The effect of most of these factors is not well understood. However, researchers have shown that oral contraceptives and obesity cause increased cholesterol in bile; cholesterol is then more likely to precipitate, forming gallstones.

37 Correct answer—D

The deposition of bile salts in the peripheral circulation, caused by the gallstones' obstruction of bile flow, results in pruritus. Research has not documented any patients exhibiting an allergy to their gallstones. The patient's anxiety about impending surgery may increase her awareness of discomfort from the condition and lead to exaggerated scratching, causing skin irritation; however, anxiety does not cause pruritus. Biliary colic causes pain, not pruritus.

38 Correct answer—A

After performing a cholecystectomy or common bile duct exploration, the physician usually performs a cholangiogram to determine if all of the stones were removed from the biliary ducts. He injects a contrast medium through the T tube, and X-rays of the biliary duct reveal whether any obstructions remain. A cholangiogram does not identify the composition of any remaining stones or problems with the sphincter of Oddi. It does not provide access to remaining stones; if any are found, the physician uses a fiber-optic duodenoscope to enlarge the opening of the sphincter of Oddi, then extracts them with a wire basket or balloon.

39 Correct answer—C

The most conclusive laboratory test result for hepatitis A is the presence of hepatitis A virus antibodies (anti-HAV IgM) in the serum; these antibodies are present only when HAV has infected the body. Serum alanine aminotransferase (ALT) is abundant in liver tissue and released when the organ is damaged; however, because the ALT level would be elevated with all three forms of hepatitis as well as other diseases (such as cardiac disease), this result does not confirm hepatitis A. Acholic stool, which lacks bile pigment, may be caused by hepatitis or by other conditions. An elevated serum level of alkaline phosphatase, an enzyme found in the liver, bones, kidneys, intestinal lining, and placenta, may be caused by various hepatic or nonhepatic conditions; it does not confirm hepatitis A.

40 Correct answer—C

During the icteric stage (after jaundice appears), the patient with hepatitis A should remain on bed rest to promote regeneration of liver tissue; physical activity should be restricted until the patient's condition improves. The nurse should force fluids to replace fluid loss from vomiting. The physician may order vitamin K administration to aid prothrombin formation and to prevent hemorrhage. The patient may experience severe pruritus during this stage; the nurse should provide mittens to prevent abrasions from the patient's fingernails when she scratches.

41 Correct answer—B

Before discharge, the nurse should caution the patient with any type of hepatitis (A; B; non-A, non-B; or D) against ever donating blood. The virus may remain active in the serum long after the acute illness passes; donating blood could transmit the disease to the recipient. The patient should wear a medical alert bracelet, but this is true of patients with many other diseases and disorders and does not require special emphasis. Hepatitis A is not transmitted through sexual contact; therefore, using a condom during sexual intercourse is not a discharge instruction the nurse must emphasize. Hand washing before and after a bowel movement is a routine hygienic precaution that the nurse should emphasize to the patient with salmonella and typhoid, not hepatitis A.

42 Correct answer—A

Mr. D. will probably receive immune serum globulin, which provides protection against hepatitis A within 7 to 10 days of exposure. A vaccine containing hepatitis B surface antigen is used to protect high-risk groups from hepatitis B before possible exposure. The bacille Calmette-Guérin vaccine offers some protection to tuberculin-negative reactors against tuberculosis, but it has no effect on hepatitis. Tetanus toxoid does not affect hepatitis either.

43 Correct answer—B

The nurse should call the physician immediately because muscle twitching and irritatability are signs of hypocalcemia, which commonly accompanies acute pancreatitis; other signs and symptoms include tetany, jerking, and positive Trousseau's and Chvostek's signs. The hypocalcemia results from fixation of calcium by fatty acids where fat necrosis has occurred and from increased amounts of circulating glucagon, which causes increased calcium loss in the urine. Muscle twitching and irritability are not commonly caused by pain; analgesics would be inappropriate. The statement about alcohol abuse is judgmental on the nurse's part and therefore inappropriate. The patient's serum amylase level would be elevated as a result of pancreatitis, but this would not cause twitching; after calling the physician, the nurse should check the patient's serum calcium level to confirm hypocalcemia.

44 Correct answer—A

The patient may assume a sitting position with the legs flexed toward the abdomen or a side-lying, knee-chest position; both relieve pressure on the abdominal muscles, reducing pain. Lying supine with the legs extended or in the lithotomy position increases pressure on abdominal muscles, causing pain. Trendelenburg's position increases pressure on the diaphragm, impairing respiration.

45 Correct answer—B

The patient with acute pancreatitis typically is hyperglycemic because of impaired insulin secretion by the pancreas. Blood glucose is usually monitored every 4 hours during the acute stages of illness; glucose solutions are usually limited, and the physician may order I.V. insulin to keep glucose levels under 200 mg/dl. Uremia is uncommon in pancreatitis; it typically results from hypovolemia with vomiting or from hemorrhagic pancreatitis.

46 Correct answer—**D**

Meperidine (Demerol) is preferred for pain relief because it does not cause spasm of the sphincter of Oddi, an adverse effect of morphine, codeine, and acetaminophen with codeine (Tylenol #3).

47 Correct answer—**C**

As acute pancreatitis subsides, the patient's diet changes from liquids to five or six small low-fat, high-carbohydrate meals daily. Foods high in carbohydrates stimulate the pancreas less than other foods. Because pancreatitis impairs fat digestion, the patient's fat intake should be limited. Caloric intake will be low because of the limited intake of fats, which usually supply a high proportion of calories.

48 Correct answer—**C**

Bread, gelatin, and cereal are high-carbohydrate, low-fat foods. Eggs, milk, cheese, pork, bacon, and cheeseburgers are high-fat foods, which the patient should avoid. Coffee, tea, and cola contain high amounts of caffeine, which stimulates the production of pancreatic juices; the patient should avoid these beverages.

49 Correct answer—**D**

Necessary long-term dietary changes include avoiding rich and spicy foods, heavy meals, and coffee as well as using antacids to decrease the production of gastric acids, which stimulate the pancreas. Antacids are used after the acute stage of pancreatitis has passed.

50 Correct answer—**D**

When establishing a behavior modification program, the nurse sets the guidelines, such as deciding to grant privileges to the patient for accomplishments; allowing the patient to set the rules does not cause a change in her behavior. Because the program is based on positive reinforcement, the nurse should avoid acting as a warden and planning a strict schedule, which the patient may view as punishment.

51 Correct answer—**D**

Although leisure time, social activity, birth weight and length, and previous illness may play a role in the development of obesity, an extremely high correlation exists between obesity in parents and children related to food intake, habits, and genetics.

52 Correct answer—D

When dieting, the patient should eat regularly spaced meals; skipping meals may only increase the tendency to eat more at the next meal. Eating slowly gives a feeling of satiety. Decreasing the size of portions helps prevent overeating. When snacks are not readily available, patients tend to eat less.

53 Correct answer—C

Valsalva's maneuver, in which the patient bears down with his mouth closed while holding his breath, increases the patient's intrathoracic pressure, preventing the introduction of air into the venous system during the normal inspiration phase. Panting would not prevent an air embolus because the patient would not be holding his breath. Ballottement is a palpatory technique used to detect an object in a fluid-filled cavity. An isometric maneuver occurs when a muscle becomes tense while remaining the same length, without movement of the joints; it would not affect the formation of an air embolus during total parenteral nutrition (TPN) catheter insertion.

54 Correct answer—B

The nurse should administer no medications, blood, or blood products through the TPN line because of possible incompatibilities between those products and any residue of the TPN solution. TPN tubing should be changed every 24 hours under strict aseptic conditions, not as needed. The Centers for Disease Control recommends dressing changes every 48 hours, not once a week. The nurse should take vital signs every 8 hours, rather than 12 hours, to monitor for temperature spikes that might indicate infection.

55 Correct answer—D

A dislodged central venous catheter causes subcutaneous emphysema, resulting in facial edema; because the catheter is located in the vena cava or right atrium, shoulder pain also is present. Rebound hypoglycemia is caused by persistent levels of insulin with interrupted administration of a hypertonic solution; glucose levels decline, resulting in hypoglycemia. Diuresis (increased urination) may be related to overly rapid infusion of a hyperosmolar solution. Muscle spasms may indicate hypoglycemia or an electrolyte balance resulting from the type of fluid administered.

56 Correct answer—A

The nurse should select foods that are chemically and mechanically nonirritating and are high in calories, protein, and minerals to restore normal nutritional levels. Foods should be nutritionally balanced, residue-free, and low-fat so they can be digested in the upper jejunum. All foods should be introduced slowly, and they should be high in protein. Certain fluids, such as cocoa and carbonated drinks, should be excluded because they tend to irritate the bowel.

57 Correct answer—D

Suction should be available or accessible for the patient receiving tube feedings to allow for immediate intervention in case of aspiration. Aspirating the residue determines how much residue remains and whether the risk of regurgitation and aspiration is increased, but this serves no purpose once aspiration occurs. Residual feedings should be reinstilled to prevent fluid and electrolyte imbalance; however, if the color or consistency is abnormal, the nurse should alert the physician and obtain a specimen. The patient should be allowed to lie on his right side, not his left, to encourage gastric emptying rather than delay it and to prevent regurgitation and aspiration.

58 Correct answer—A

The nurse must assess for dehydration in the patient receiving tube feedings, because fluid loss may result from excessive diarrhea, excessive protein intake, or osmotic diuresis. Osmotic diuresis may result from a high glucose load when the rate of infusion has been increased, not decreased. Although lethargy and disorientation indicate fluid volume deficit, engorged neck veins indicate fluid overload. Immobility and low-residual feedings may cause constipation, but they are more likely to cause diarrhea because hyperosmolar feedings require the addition of water to the formula.

59 Correct answer—D

The patient should observe for signs of electrolyte imbalance (including poor skin turgor, muscle weakness, and restlessness or lethargy) or bacterial infection (including abdominal distention, cramps, or diarrhea) and report any such signs at once; this helps prevent further complications. The formula should be at room temperature before administration begins, not ends; cold formula may cause abdominal cramps. Tube patency should be checked before each feeding by instilling a small amount of water. The patient should position himself to prevent aspiration, not increase his comfort; usually, his head is elevated at least 30 degrees.

CHAPTER 5

Renal
System

Questions

1 Which nursing intervention would best prevent acute renal failure in the postsurgical patient?

A. Having the patient deep-breathe and cough every hour to prevent lung congestion
B. Taking vital signs every 2 hours to identify impending hemorrhage and shock
C. Turning the patient every 2 hours to promote venous return to the heart
D. Monitoring I.V. fluids every 4 hours to prevent fluid overload

2 Which action should the nurse take when caring for a patient in the oliguric phase of acute renal failure?

A. Encouraging a low-carbohydrate diet
B. Observing for signs and symptoms of osteodystrophy
C. Helping the patient maintain fluid restrictions
D. Encouraging increased ambulation

3 The physician orders aluminum hydroxide (Amphojel) with each meal for a patient with end-stage renal disease. This drug is given to:

A. Remove protein wastes of metabolism
B. Bind phosphorus in the GI tract
C. Exchange sodium for potassium in the colon
D. Inhibit development of a stress ulcer

4 Which finding indicates potassium toxicity in a patient with end-stage renal disease?

A. Bilateral crackles
B. Elevated temperature
C. Chvostek's sign
D. Muscle weakness and paresthesia

5 Which outcome should the nurse expect after peritoneal dialysis?

A. Decreased serum urea nitrogen concentration
B. Stimulated urine formation from external kidney pressure
C. Increased serum glucose concentration
D. Removal of excess serum parathyroid hormone

6 Mr. Q., a patient undergoing peritoneal dialysis, experiences shortness of breath. Which action should the nurse take first?

A. Elevating the head of the bed and observing the patient
B. Slowing the instillation of the dialyzing solution
C. Checking the patient's vital signs and weight and documenting the findings
D. Draining the fluid from the peritoneal cavity and notifying the physician

7 Cyclosporine (Sandimmune) is used to prevent kidney transplant rejection. The toxic effects of cyclosporine do *not* include:

A. Nephrotoxicity
B. Splenomegaly
C. Bone marrow depression
D. Hirsutism

8 Before a kidney transplant, the nurse should *not* tell the donor that:

A. One kidney will maintain adequate renal function
B. His position during surgery will cause muscle aches and pain
C. The physician will make an incision in the flank area
D. He will require 3 months of immunosuppressant therapy after surgery

9 Which patient would have the lowest proportion of fluid volume to body weight?

A. A 65-year-old man
B. A 7-month-old boy
C. A muscular 26-year-old man
D. An obese 45-year-old woman

10 The adrenal glands control fluid and electrolyte balance primarily by:

A. Producing antidiuretic hormone
B. Stimulating osmoreceptors
C. Secreting glucocorticoids and mineralocorticoids
D. Secreting catecholamines

11 Which type of solution causes water to shift from the cells into the plasma?

A. Hypertonic
B. Hypotonic
C. Isotonic
D. Alkaline

12 Particles move from an area of greater osmolality to one of lesser osmolality through:

A. Active transport
B. Osmosis
C. Diffusion
D. Filtration

13 Which solution is *not* considered isotonic?

A. Dextrose 5% in water
B. Lactated Ringer's solution
C. Normal saline solution
D. Dextrose 5% in half-normal saline solution

14 Which assessment finding indicates dehydration?

A. "Tenting" of chest skin when pinched
B. Rapid filling of hand veins
C. A pulse that is not easily obliterated
D. Neck vein distention

15 Which laboratory test result is *not* common in a patient with water intoxication?

A. A low hemoglobin level
B. A low hematocrit
C. A low urine specific gravity
D. An elevated serum sodium level

16 Which nursing intervention would most likely lead to a hypo-osmolar state?

A. Performing nasogastric tube irrigation with normal saline solution
B. Weighing the patient daily
C. Administering tap water enemas until return is clear
D. Encouraging a patient with excessive perspiration to drink broth

17 The major extracellular buffering system, essential in maintaining normal pH, depends on:

A. Plasma protein
B. The bicarbonate–carbonic acid ratio
C. Blood phosphates
D. Renal secretion of ammonia

18 Which condition is indicated by a pH of 7.16, a partial pressure of carbon dioxide in arterial blood of 75 mm Hg, a bicarbonate level of 25 mEq/liter, a partial pressure of oxygen in arterial blood of 69 mm Hg, and a base excess of –3 mEq/liter?

A. Respiratory acidosis
B. Compensated respiratory acidosis
C. Metabolic acidosis
D. Compensated metabolic acidosis

19 Treatment for a patient with acute pancreatitis and hypocalcemia should include administration of calcium supplements and:

A. Potassium supplements
B. Packed red blood cells
C. Vitamin D (Deltalin)
D. Furosemide (Lasix)

20 Nursing assessment of a patient in metabolic alkalosis resulting from chronic alcohol abuse would reveal all of the following findings *except:*

A. Nausea and vomiting
B. Belligerence and irritability
C. Decreased thoracic movement
D. Positive Chvostek's sign

21 Which assessment finding would indicate an extracellular fluid volume deficit?

A. Bradycardia
B. A central venous pressure of 6 mm Hg
C. Pitting edema
D. An orthostatic blood pressure change

22 Which type of fluid shift is indicated by 2+ pitting edema and severe ascites in a patient with advanced cirrhosis of the liver?

A. Extracellular to intracellular
B. Intracellular to extracellular
C. Interstitial space to plasma
D. Plasma to interstitial space

SITUATION

Mr. P., a 60-year-old architect, is admitted to the hospital with benign prostatic hyperplasia (BPH).

Questions 23 to 27 refer to this situation.

23 Nursing assessment of the patient with BPH would most likely reveal:

A. Dysuria, urinary hesitancy, and dribbling
B. Flank pain and decreased caliber of urine stream
C. Urinary frequency, nocturia, and decreased force of urine stream
D. Hematuria, urinary hesitancy, and pyuria

24 The physician inserts an indwelling urinary (Foley) catheter to relieve Mr. P.'s urine retention. Which nursing action would *not* help maintain the drainage system's patency?

A. Taping the catheter to the inner aspect of the thigh
B. Forcing fluids (more than 3,000 ml/day)
C. Keeping the drainage bag below the bladder level
D. Positioning the tubing without dependent loops

25 The physician schedules Mr. P. for a transurethral resection of the prostate (TURP) under spinal anesthesia. Before surgery, the nurse should tell the patient that:

A. He may receive continuous bladder irrigation after the procedure
B. The procedure may cause impotency
C. Sterility is a common complication of this procedure
D. The physician will remove the entire prostate during this procedure

26 Because of the position Mr. P. must assume during TURP, the nurse should assess him postoperatively for:

A. Incision site infection
B. Thrombophlebitis
C. Atelectasis
D. Water intoxication

27 The fourth day after the procedure, the physician removes Mr. P.'s indwelling urinary (Foley) catheter. Later that day, he complains of "wetting" his pajamas to the nurse. Which nursing intervention is most appropriate?

A. Advising the patient to contract his perineal muscles periodically
B. Restricting his fluid intake
C. Applying a condom catheter
D. Suggesting that the patient void as soon as the urge occurs

SITUATION

Mrs. Y., a 35-year-old homemaker, is admitted with signs and symptoms of urinary tract infection.

Questions 28 and 29 refer to this situation.

28 Mrs. Y.'s physician diagnoses acute pyelonephritis. Which clinical manifestations should the nurse expect?

A. Lower abdominal pain, dysuria, and urinary frequency
B. Pyuria, hematuria, and groin pain
C. Flank pain, urinary frequency, and an elevated white blood cell (WBC) count
D. Urinary frequency and casts in the urine

29 The physician orders a combination of sulfisoxazole and phenazopyridine hydrochloride (Azo Gantrisin) for Mrs. Y. Which therapeutic effect should this combination drug have?

A. Pain relief and a decreased WBC count
B. Equal fluid intake and output
C. Polyuria with a reddish stain
D. Increased complaints of bladder spasm after 20 minutes

SITUATION

Mrs. J., age 50, is admitted to the hospital for cystoscopic examination to assess for bladder cancer. Cystoscopy confirms the diagnosis. After inserting an indwelling urinary (Foley) catheter, Mrs. J.'s physician orders chemotherapy with doxorubicin (Adriamycin RDF) and thiotepa and schedules her for a cystectomy with ileal conduit urinary diversion.

Questions 30 to 32 refer to this situation.

---

30 The most common early sign of bladder tumors is:

A. Painless hematuria
B. A change in voiding pattern
C. Abrupt weight gain
D. Weakness

---

31 The purpose of Mrs. J.'s chemotherapy is to:

A. Eliminate the need for surgery
B. Augment the treatment regimen
C. Reduce pain and anxiety before surgery
D. Sterilize the bowel before surgery

---

32 Which topic should *not* be reviewed by the nurse during Mrs. J.'s preoperative patient-teaching session?

A. The patient's ability to describe the surgical procedure
B. The patient's knowledge that the procedure creates a stoma and that she must wear a pouch afterward
C. The patient's need to perform stoma care immediately after surgery to ensure mastering self-care before discharge
D. The patient's understanding that her physical activities, work, hobbies, and clothing style need not change after surgery

---

SITUATION

Mrs. G., a 34-year-old homemaker, is admitted to the hospital with a diagnosis of renal calculi.

Questions 33 to 35 refer to this situation.

33 Which factor does *not* predispose an individual to renal calculi development?

A. A history of urinary tract infections
B. Prolonged immobilization
C. Hyperkalemia
D. Hypervitaminosis D

34 Clinical manifestations of renal calculi depend on all of the following factors *except:*

A. The composition of the calculi
B. The site of the calculi
C. The degree of obstruction
D. The presence of infection

35 The results of Mrs. G.'s blood studies show a blood urea nitrogen (BUN) level of 20 mg/dl, serum calcium level of 4.5 mEq/liter, serum phosphorus level of 1.8 mEq/liter, serum sodium level of 138 mEq/liter, and urine pH of 5.1. Which nursing intervention would be most effective in altering Mrs. G.'s urine pH?

A. Increasing activity
B. Forcing fluids
C. Administering allopurinol (Zyloprim) as ordered
D. Excluding high-calcium foods from her diet

SITUATION

Mrs. O., age 50, is admitted to the unit with a diagnosis of chronic glomerulonephritis.

Questions 36 to 40 refer to this situation.

36 Characteristic clinical manifestations of chronic glomerulonephritis include:

A. A blood pressure over 130/85 mm Hg
B. A BUN level over 60 mg/dl
C. Slightly swollen joints
D. Apprehension

37 Mrs. O. mentions that she likes salty foods. The nurse should instruct her to lower her sodium intake to:

A. Promote urea nitrogen excretion
B. Improve her glomerular filtration rate
C. Increase potassium absorption
D. Reduce edema

38 Before Mrs. O.'s discharge, the nurse should teach her about the need for:

A. A nephrectomy
B. A high-protein diet
C. Protection from infections
D. Foot care

39 Two months later, Mrs. O. is readmitted with renal failure. After efforts to reverse Mrs. O.'s condition are unsuccessful, the physician creates an arteriovenous fistula in her left arm for dialysis. Which nursing measure is necessary to maintain the fistula?

A. Instructing the patient not to exercise her arm
B. Avoiding blood pressure measurements in the left arm
C. Observing for cannula separation at the connection site
D. Applying a dry, sterile dressing daily

40 Which observation involving Mrs. O.'s fistula would require the nurse to notify the physician?

A. Blood flow detected while palpating the fistula site
B. Blood flow observed through the cannula
C. Absence of an audible bruit while auscultating the graft
D. Straw-colored blood flow observed through the cannula

SITUATION

Mr. D., age 45, is admitted to the emergency department (ED) in metabolic acidosis caused by an aspirin overdose.

Questions 41 and 42 refer to this situation.

41 Which assessment finding would *not* be a clinical manifestation of metabolic acidosis?

A. Confusion
B. Vomiting
C. Hypoventilation
D. Lethargy

42 To prevent potential complications in Mr. D., the nurse should:

A. Administer oxygen continuously
B. Insert an indwelling urinary (Foley) catheter
C. Prepare the patient for hemodialysis
D. Prepare 10% calcium gluconate for administration

SITUATION

Mr. L., age 40, is admitted to the hospital in uncompensated respiratory acidosis caused by a spontaneous pneumothorax.

Questions 43 and 44 refer to this situation.

43 Which arterial blood gas values indicate uncompensated respiratory acidosis?

A. pH of 7.32, partial pressure of carbon dioxide in arterial blood ($PaCO_2$) of 60 mm Hg, and bicarbonate (HCO_3^-) level of 39 mEq/liter
B. pH of 7.18, $PaCO_2$ of 64 mm Hg, and HCO_3^- level of 24 mEq/liter
C. pH of 7.18, $PaCO_2$ of 34 mm Hg, and HCO_3^- level of 19 mEq/liter
D. pH of 7.50, $PaCO_2$ of 25 mm Hg, and HCO_3^- level of 24 mEq/liter

44 Mr. L.'s body will attempt to compensate for this acid-base imbalance by:

A. Increasing the formation and excretion of ammonia ions
B. Moving potassium into the cells in exchange for hydrogen and sodium
C. Decreasing the rate and depth of respirations
D. Increasing HCO_3^- excretion by the kidneys

SITUATION

Mrs. G., age 28, is admitted to the ED after a house fire. She has second- and third-degree burns over approximately 30% of her body surface area (BSA).

Questions 45 to 48 refer to this situation.

---

45 Which parenteral solution should Mrs. G. receive during the fluid resuscitation phase of her treatment?

A. Dextrose 5% in water
B. Lactated Ringer's solution
C. Hypotonic saline solution
D. 20 mEq of potassium chloride in half-normal saline solution

---

46 Which information is *not* used when the nurse calculates and maintains Mrs. G.'s I.V. therapy for fluid resuscitation?

A. Depth and BSA percentage of burns
B. Sex and past medical history
C. Hematocrit and hemoglobin values
D. Urine output and specific gravity

---

47 Which fluid and electrolyte imbalances are likely to occur in the initial stage of Mrs. G.'s burn injury?

A. Interstitial-to-plasma fluid shift and sodium excess
B. Plasma-to-interstitial fluid shift and potassium excess
C. Interstitial-to-extracellular fluid shift and sodium deficit
D. Intracellular-to-intravascular fluid shift and potassium deficit

---

48 Which laboratory value indicates that Mrs. G.'s water intake should be restricted?

A. Elevated serum sodium level
B. Elevated serum potassium level
C. Decreased serum sodium level
D. Decreased serum magnesium level

SITUATION

Mr. E., a 40-year-old teacher, is admitted to the hospital with lethargy and tachypnea. His skin is dry and flushed, and his breath has a fruity odor. His blood glucose level is 840 mg/dl; urinalysis reveals +3 glucose and +3 ketones. The physician diagnoses diabetic ketoacidosis (DKA).

Questions 49 and 50 refer to this situation.

49 DKA causes all of the following assessment findings *except:*

A. Hypo-osmolality
B. Dehydration
C. Hyperkalemia
D. Hypocapnia

50 Which I.V. solution would probably be used in Mr. E.'s initial treatment?

A. Isotonic saline solution
B. Hypotonic saline solution
C. Hypertonic saline solution
D. Lactated Ringer's solution

SITUATION

Mrs. T., age 78, is admitted to the unit with a chief complaint of abdominal cramping. She states that she has had diarrhea and has felt tired for about a week. She has a past medical history of diabetes mellitus and chronic renal failure. Her serum potassium level is 6 mEq/liter, indicating hyperkalemia.

Questions 51 to 53 refer to this situation.

51 Pharmacologic management of Mrs. T.'s hyperkalemia may include all of the following measures *except:*

A. Lactulose (Chronulac) enemas
B. Glucose and insulin I.V.
C. Sodium bicarbonate I.V.
D. Calcium chloride I.V.

52 Physical assessment of Mrs. T. would probably reveal:

A. Oliguria and apathy
B. Tetany
C. Bradypnea
D. Hyperactive bowel sounds and polyuria

53 Which acid-base abnormality commonly is associated with hyperkalemia?

A. Respiratory acidosis
B. Metabolic alkalosis
C. Respiratory alkalosis
D. Metabolic acidosis

SITUATION

Mr. F., age 48, complains of fatigue, weakness, and palpitations. After several diagnostic tests, the physician determines that these symptoms are caused by hypophosphatemia.

Questions 54 to 56 refer to this situation.

---

54 The most common cause of hypophosphatemia is:

A. Acute renal failure
B. Chronic alcoholism
C. Alkalosis
D. Chronic renal failure

---

55 Assessment of Mr. F. most likely would reveal:

A. Numbness around the mouth
B. Clinical manifestations of hypercalcemia
C. Carpopedal spasm
D. Muscle twitching and cramping

---

56 Mr. F.'s initial treatment should include the administration of:

A. Potassium phosphate (Neutra-Phos-K)
B. Acetazolamide (Diamox)
C. Aluminum hydroxide (Amphojel)
D. Vitamins

Answer sheet

	A	B	C	D			A	B	C	D
1	○	○	○	○		31	○	○	○	○
2	○	○	○	○		32	○	○	○	○
3	○	○	○	○		33	○	○	○	○
4	○	○	○	○		34	○	○	○	○
5	○	○	○	○		35	○	○	○	○
6	○	○	○	○		36	○	○	○	○
7	○	○	○	○		37	○	○	○	○
8	○	○	○	○		38	○	○	○	○
9	○	○	○	○		39	○	○	○	○
10	○	○	○	○		40	○	○	○	○
11	○	○	○	○		41	○	○	○	○
12	○	○	○	○		42	○	○	○	○
13	○	○	○	○		43	○	○	○	○
14	○	○	○	○		44	○	○	○	○
15	○	○	○	○		45	○	○	○	○
16	○	○	○	○		46	○	○	○	○
17	○	○	○	○		47	○	○	○	○
18	○	○	○	○		48	○	○	○	○
19	○	○	○	○		49	○	○	○	○
20	○	○	○	○		50	○	○	○	○
21	○	○	○	○		51	○	○	○	○
22	○	○	○	○		52	○	○	○	○
23	○	○	○	○		53	○	○	○	○
24	○	○	○	○		54	○	○	○	○
25	○	○	○	○		55	○	○	○	○
26	○	○	○	○		56	○	○	○	○
27	○	○	○	○						
28	○	○	○	○						
29	○	○	○	○						
30	○	○	○	○						

Answers and rationales

1 Correct answer—**B**

Unresolved shock from hemorrhage leads to decreased vascular volume; this causes inadequate hydrostatic pressure for glomerular filtration, resulting in renal failure. Lung congestion is not a complication of postoperative renal failure. Turning the patient every 2 hours prevents embolism, not renal failure. Fluid overload is a result, not a cause, of renal failure.

2 Correct answer—**C**

The nurse should help the patient maintain fluid restrictions. The degree of restriction varies depending on kidney output; only enough fluids to replace losses is allowed. Carbohydrates, an essential nutrient, are not restricted; if carbohydrate intake is inadequate, the body metabolizes protein for energy. Osteodystrophy is a complication of end-stage renal disease, not acute renal failure. Bed rest is recommended to conserve energy, reduce the metabolic rate, and decrease edema; ambulation should be restricted during the early oliguric stage.

3 Correct answer—**B**

Aluminum hydroxide (Amphojel) is given to control serum phosphorus; this drug neutralizes gastric acidity and binds with phosphates in the GI tract to increase phosphorus excretion. With chronic renal failure, unfiltered waste products of metabolism, such as protein, accumulate in the blood; however, aluminum hydroxide has no effect on the excretion of protein or other waste products. This drug does not exchange sodium for potassium; sodium polystyrene sulfonate (Kayexalate) has this effect. End-stage renal disease does not necessarily lead to a stress ulcer; in addition, antacids do not inhibit ulcers but reduce gastric acidity, which increases with a peptic ulcer.

4 Correct answer—**D**

Potassium, an intracellular cation, is necessary for neuromuscular function; muscle weakness and paresthesia are symptoms of hyperkalemia, a common complication of end-stage renal disease. Bilateral crackles are caused by various conditions, such as congestive heart failure, and are not typically associated with end-stage renal disease. An elevated temperature is not related to potassium toxicity. A positive Chvostek's sign indicates hypocalcemia, not hyperkalemia.

5 Correct answer—A

The nurse should expect a decreased serum urea nitrogen concentration after peritoneal dialysis, a procedure that removes waste products from the body when the kidneys are not functioning properly. Although the instillation of fluid into the peritoneal cavity increases intra-abdominal pressure, peritoneal dialysis does not stimulate urine formation, nor does it affect the level of serum glucose or parathyroid hormone.

6 Correct answer—A

The nurse's first action should be to elevate the head of the bed and observe the patient for improved breathing; elevating the patient's head reduces the pressure on the diaphragm caused by fluid accumulation in the abdomen, which can cause shortness of breath. Because slowing the instillation would not greatly reduce pressure on the thorax, this action would not help the patient's breathing. Checking vital signs and weight and documenting these findings provides data, but this situation calls for immediate nursing intervention. Draining the fluid and notifying the physician would not be necessary initially if elevating the patient's head improves breathing; if circulatory overload is causing the problem instead, the nurse should call the physician.

7 Correct answer—C

Bone marrow depression is not a toxic effect of cyclosporine; it is a major toxic effect of the immunosuppressant azathioprine (Imuran). Nephrotoxicity, splenomegaly, and hirsutism are possible toxic effects of cyclosporine.

8 Correct answer—D

A kidney donor is treated like any postnephrectomy patient; immunosuppressant drugs are not used because the donor is not receiving the transplant. However, the donor should be reassured about the ability of the remaining kidney to maintain adequate renal function. The nurse should also inform the donor that his position during surgery will cause some muscle pain and that the physician will make a flank incision.

9 Correct answer—D

An obese 45-year-old woman would have the lowest proportion of fluid volume to body weight. Percentage of total body fluid varies with age, sex, and amount of total body fat, which is almost entirely water-free. In infants, fluid accounts for about 80% of body weight; this percentage steadily decreases with age. By adulthood, body fluid accounts for about 60% of a normal lean man's body weight; because women have proportionately more fat than men, body fluid accounts for 45% to 50% of a normal lean woman's weight. At age 60, the percentage drops to 45% for both men and women.

10 Correct answer—C

The adrenal glands control fluid and electrolyte balance primarily by secreting mineralocorticoids and glucocorticoids. Aldosterone, the principal mineralocorticoid, increases sodium reabsorption and potassium excretion. Glucocorticoids also affect water balance, but the exact mechanism is uncertain; it may be related to glucose levels creating an osmotic pull. Although antidiuretic hormone (ADH) does affect water retention, it is secreted by the posterior pituitary gland, not the adrenal glands. When osmoreceptors are stimulated by high sodium levels resulting from increased aldosterone levels, they increase secretion of ADH from the posterior pituitary gland. The adrenal medulla secretes the catecholamines epinephrine, norepinephrine, and dopamine, but they do not directly affect fluid and electrolyte balance.

11 Correct answer—A

A hypertonic solution causes water to shift from the cells into the plasma because the solution has a greater osmotic pressure than the cells. A hypotonic solution has a lower osmotic pressure than that of the cells; it causes fluid to shift into the cells, possibly resulting in rupture. An isotonic solution, which has the same osmotic pressure as the cells, would not cause any shift. A solution's alkalinity is related to its hydrogen ion concentration, not its osmotic effect.

12 Correct answer—C

Particles move from an area of greater osmolality to one of lesser osmolality through diffusion, the random movement of particles in a solution toward uniform distribution from brownian (thermal) movement. Active transport is the movement of particles through energy expenditure from other sources, such as enzymes. Osmosis is the movement of a pure solvent through a semipermeable membrane from an area of greater osmolality to one of lesser osmolality until equalization occurs; the membrane is impermeable to the solute but permeable to the solvent. Filtration is the process by which fluid is forced through a membrane by a difference in pressure; small molecules pass through, but large ones do not.

13 Correct answer—D

An isotonic solution has nearly the same osmolality as serum, which is normally 275 to 300 mOsm/kg of water; the osmolality of dextrose 5% in half-normal saline solution is 406 mOsm/kg of water. Dextrose 5% in water has an osmolality of 252 mOsm/kg of water; lactated Ringer's solution, 273 mOsm/kg of water; and normal saline solution, 308 mOsm/kg of water.

14 Correct answer—A

Tenting of chest skin when pinched indicates dehydration; because of the decrease in skin elasticity, pinching the skin causes an indentation called tenting or inverted V. Hand veins fill slowly with dehydration, not rapidly. A pulse that is not easily obliterated and neck vein distention indicate fluid overload, not dehydration.

15 Correct answer—D

An elevated sodium level is not common in a patient with water intoxication; because sodium is diluted from excess fluid, the sodium level typically is low. Because of hemodilution, the hemoglobin level and hematocrit commonly are low; urine specific gravity is low from dilution.

16 Correct answer—C

Administering a tap water enema until return is clear would most likely contribute to a hypo-osmolar state; because tap water is hypotonic, it would be absorbed by the body, diluting the body fluid concentration and lowering osmolarity. Some institutions use commercial hypertonic enemas containing sodium to prevent this; others have standing orders to clean the colon with polyethylene glycol-electrolyte solution (GoLYTELY), which contains sodium, potassium, and bicarbonate. Both methods cause less fluid and electrolyte shifting. Weighing the patient is the easiest, most accurate method to determine fluid changes; it helps identify—rather than contribute to—a fluid imbalance. Nasogastric tube irrigation with normal saline solution, an isotonic solution, would not cause a shift in fluid balance. Drinking broth would not contribute to a hypo-osmolar state because it does not replace sodium and water lost through excessive perspiration.

17 Correct answer—B

The major extracellular buffering system depends on the bicarbonate–carbonic acid ratio. The normal ratio to maintain acid-base balance is 1 carbonic acid molecule to 20 sodium bicarbonate molecules. The respiratory system and kidneys regulate these two elements; the respiratory system eliminates excess carbon dioxide and water, and the kidneys conserve or eliminate bicarbonate. Plasma protein and blood phosphates exert an intracellular buffering effect by converting strong acids to neutral salts or strong bases to water. Renal secretion of ammonia is not part of the buffering system, although ammonia combines with and eliminates excess hydrogen ions in the kidney tubules.

18 Correct answer—A

These arterial blood gas levels indicate respiratory acidosis. The pH is lower than normal (7.35 to 7.45), indicating a high hydrogen ion concentration, or acidosis. The partial pressure of carbon dioxide in arterial blood ($PaCO_2$) is above normal (35 to 45 mm Hg), which indicates a respiratory disorder rather than a metabolic one. The bicarbonate (HCO_3^-) value is within the normal range (22 to 26 mm Hg). Because the body normally tries to compensate for an acute acid-base imbalance, this normal value indicates that no compensation has occurred yet. Compensation consists of noncausative factor changes in the opposite direction of the abnormal pH; with acute respiratory acidosis, the HCO_3^- value normally would rise by 1 mEq/liter for every increase of 10 mm Hg in $PaCO_2$ if the body were compensating for the imbalance.

19 Correct answer—C

Along with calcium supplementation, treatment should include daily administration of vitamin D (Deltalin), which is essential for calcium absorption. Potassium supplementation is not necessary; because potassium and calcium do not have a reciprocal relationship, potassium supplements would have no effect on hypocalcemia. Packed red blood cells would not improve the patient's condition either. Furosemide (Lasix) is used to treat hypercalcemia, not hypocalcemia.

20 Correct answer—A

A patient in metabolic alkalosis would not demonstrate nausea and vomiting; this finding is associated with acidosis. The rising pH causes stimulation of the central nervous system, resulting in belligerence and irritability. Decreased thoracic movement and shallow respirations also would be present as the body attempts to compensate by conserving carbon dioxide. High pH also increases protein binding of calcium, causing hypocalcemia; Chvostek's sign would be positive.

21 Correct answer—D

An orthostatic blood pressure change indicates an extracellular fluid volume deficit. The extracellular compartment comprises both the intravascular compartment and interstitial space. A fluid volume deficit within the intravascular compartment would cause tachycardia, not bradycardia, and orthostatic blood pressure changes. To confirm this, the nurse should take the patient's blood pressure while he is lying down, then again while he is sitting up. A drop of 15 mm Hg or more in systolic pressure or of 10 mm Hg or more in diastolic pressure indicates an orthostatic change. A central venous pressure of 6 mm Hg is in the high normal range, indicating adequate hydration. Pitting edema indicates fluid volume overload.

22 Correct answer—D

The patient's assessment findings indicate a fluid shift from the plasma to interstitial space. Advanced cirrhosis typically results in portal hypertension; the increased pressure leads to transudation of sodium and fluid into the peritoneal cavity, causing ascites. Oncotic (colloidal osmotic) pressure drops because of poor protein intake and synthesis. This allows protein-rich fluid to shift from the plasma to interstitial space, causing edema.

23 Correct answer—C

Urinary frequency, nocturia, and decreased force and caliber of the urine stream are common clinical manifestations of BPH; they result from urethral obstruction. Dysuria, urinary hesitancy, dribbling, and pyuria are associated with irritation, possibly from infection. Flank pain is common with kidney inflammation, not BPH. Hematuria indicates cancer of the prostate, not BPH.

24 Correct answer—A

Taping an indwelling urinary (Foley) catheter to the inner aspect of the thigh would prevent tension on the urinary meatus; it would not help maintain the drainage system's patency. Forcing fluids maintains urine volume, causing steady movement of urine through the drainage system and preventing blood clot formation. Keeping the drainage bag below bladder level also allows steady drainage from gravity. Preventing dependent loops helps prevent drainage stagnation, which may cause an obstruction in the system from debris.

25 Correct answer—A

Continuous bladder irrigation is common after transurethral resection of the prostate (TURP); it promotes the removal of blood clots from the bladder. Impotency is a potential complication with perineal prostatic resection, not TURP. Because the testes are not removed during this procedure, sterility is uncommon. The physician does not remove the entire prostate during TURP.

26 Correct answer—B

Thrombophlebitis is a potential complication after TURP because the patient must assume the lithotomy position for a prolonged period; this causes pressure at the popliteal area, which may lead to venous stasis and resulting thrombophlebitis. Incision site infection is not a potential complication of this procedure because of an absence of an open incision site. Atelectasis is not a common complication of TURP; it is more likely after a perineal prostatectomy or a procedure requiring inhalational general anesthetics. Water intoxication may result from continuous bladder irrigation during the procedure, but this complication is not related to the patient's position.

27 Correct answer—A

Perineal muscle contraction helps reestablish bladder sphincter tone and control voiding. Unless contraindicated, fluids should be forced, not restricted, after TURP to maintain renal function. Applying a condom catheter will prevent soiling, but it will not reestablish sphincter control. Stopping and starting the urine stream would be more effective in reestablishing sphincter control than voiding when the urge occurs.

28 Correct answer—C

Flank pain, urinary frequency, and an elevated white blood cell (WBC) count are common clinical manifestations of pyelonephritis. Lower abdominal pain, dysuria, urinary frequency, and groin pain are associated with cystitis. Pyuria, hematuria, and casts in the urine are common with glomerulonephritis.

29 Correct answer—A

This combination drug's therapeutic effects include pain relief and a decreased WBC count; phenazopyridine is an analgesic, and sulfisoxazole is an antibiotic. The drug does not affect fluid intake or output; however, because sulfisoxazole is a sulfa preparation, the patient's fluid intake should be increased to prevent crystallization in the urine. The drug does cause a reddish stain in the urine, but this effect has no therapeutic value. The patient's complaints of bladder spasm should decrease, not increase, after administration of this drug.

30 Correct answer—A

Painless hematuria is the first clinical manifestation in most patients with bladder tumors. A change in voiding pattern commonly results from renal failure or prostate enlargement. Abrupt weight gain is caused by fluid retention, a symptom of renal failure or cardiac failure. Weakness is a nonspecific symptom of many disorders; it is not commonly seen with bladder tumors.

31 Correct answer—B

Chemotherapy augments the patient's treatment regimen; it destroys tumor cells before surgical removal of the tumor, reducing the risk that cancer may spread or recur. Chemotherapy in bladder cancer typically is not curative; it does not eliminate the need for surgery. The chemotherapeutic agents doxorubicin (Adriamycin RDF) and thiotepa have no analgesic or sedative actions; they do not reduce pain or anxiety. Bowel sterilization is not necessary before a cystectomy.

32 Correct answer—C

The nurse will perform stoma care immediately after surgery, and the patient will assist to help master self-care before discharge. Knowledge of the surgical procedure is necessary to obtain an informed consent. The patient should be aware that she will have a stoma and that she must wear a pouch after the procedure. The nurse should demonstrate urostomy appliances and how they adhere to the body without hindering physical activities, work, hobbies, or clothing style.

33 Correct answer—C

Hyperkalemia is not a predisposing factor for renal calculi formation. Stone formation follows the precipitation of minerals around organic nuclei, such as bacteria, blood clots, and dead tissue; these minerals include calcium oxalate, calcium phosphate, magnesium ammonium phosphate, uric acid, and cystine, but not potassium. Urinary tract infections increase the amount of organic material around which calculi may form. Prolonged immobilization leads to loss of bone calcium, and hypervitaminosis D increases calcium absorption from the intestines; with both conditions, the excessive calcium in the bloodstream may adhere to organic material and form calculi.

34 Correct answer—A

The composition of renal calculi does not affect clinical manifestations, although the information may indicate possible causes; for example, calcium stones—the most common type—may be caused by prolonged immobility, excessive intake of vitamin D, malabsorption syndrome, and altered renal reabsorption of calcium. The site of the calculi, degree of obstruction, and presence of infection influence the clinical manifestations exhibited. For example, stones in ureters may cause colicky pain radiating down the thigh; obstruction may cause pain and hydronephrosis; and urinary tract infection, commonly resulting from stones in the bladder, may cause chills, fever, and dysuria.

35 Correct answer—C

The most effective nursing intervention to alter this patient's urine pH would be administering allopurinol (Zyloprim) as ordered; allopurinol decreases uric acid levels by inhibiting conversion of xanthine oxidase to uric acid, which results in more alkaline urine. Increased activity would increase peristalsis, helping to propel the stone downward and out if it is not a staghorn calculus; however, it would not affect the urine pH. Forcing fluids would help flush urates from the kidney and prevent crystallization of more stones, but it would not affect the urine pH. Excluding high-calcium foods would not affect urine pH and would only decrease the formation of stones composed of calcium salts, not of stones composed of other minerals.

36 Correct answer—B

The normal blood urea nitrogen (BUN) level is 6 to 20 mg/dl; an elevated level indicates renal failure, a result of glomeruli inflammation in chronic glomerulonephritis. Because waste products from metabolic processes, such as BUN, are not filtered, excessive amounts accumulate in the blood. A blood pressure of 130/85 mm Hg is normal for a 50-year-old woman. Swollen joints are not characteristic of chronic glomerulonephritis. Apprehension is normal for a newly admitted patient; however, it is not specifically related to this disease.

37 Correct answer—D

Reducing sodium intake reduces fluid retention. Excess retained fluid increases blood volume, which changes blood vessel permeability and allows plasma to move into interstitial tissue, causing edema. Urea nitrogen excretion can be increased only by improved renal function. Sodium intake does not affect the glomerular filtration rate. Potassium absorption is improved only by increasing the glomerular filtration rate; it is not affected by sodium intake.

38 Correct answer—C

To prevent further episodes of chronic glomerulonephritis, the patient must protect herself against infections, which increase the metabolic rate and result in more waste products; their excretion is decreased because of impaired kidney function. Recurrent infections also predispose the kidneys to greater damage. Even if the patient has renal failure, a nephrectomy would not necessarily be indicated. A high-protein diet is contraindicated because of impaired removal of protein wastes. Foot problems are not associated with glomerulonephritis.

39 Correct answer—B

The nurse should not take blood pressure measurements in the left arm because this may compromise circulation to the fistula; clot formation may occur, reducing the fistula's patency or rendering it useless. The patient should exercise the arm to promote circulation through the fistula. Because the fistula is internal, the nurse would not be able to observe any separation of the cannula at the connection site. Applying a dry, sterile dressing is unnecessary once the incision has healed.

40 Correct answer—C

The nurse should hear turbulent blood flow through the vessels using the bell of the stethoscope; absence of a bruit indicates a non-patent fistula, requiring the nurse to notify the physician. Blood flow detected while palpating the fistula site indicates that the fistula is patent; notifying the physician would not be necessary. Because an arteriovenous fistula does not require an external cannula, blood flow—regardless of the color—would not be visible.

41 Correct answer—C

Hyperventilation—not hypoventilation—occurs with metabolic acidosis; the body attempts to eliminate excess carbon dioxide through deep, rapid breathing (Kussmaul's respirations). Metabolic acidosis causes central nervous system depression, resulting in confusion and lethargy. Vomiting is caused by the high concentration of hydrogen ions in the plasma.

42 Correct answer—**D**

To prevent potential complications of metabolic acidosis, the nurse should prepare 10% calcium gluconate for I.V. administration. As acidosis is corrected, pH climbs, decreasing the patient's ionized calcium concentration. The nurse should administer oxygen cautiously to provide ventilation until blood gases are drawn and discontinue it if the pH rises above 7.5. Monitoring the fluid balance to detect possible hypovolemia is essential; however, if the patient is conscious, an indwelling urinary (Foley) catheter may not be needed to monitor the urine output. Hemodialysis may be used to remove aspirin from the blood, preventing further complications, but it is not commonly needed.

43 Correct answer—**B**

A pH of 7.18, partial pressure of carbon dioxide in arterial blood ($PaCO_2$) of 64 mm Hg, and HCO_3^- level of 24 mEq/liter indicate uncompensated respiratory acidosis; the low pH and elevated $PaCO_2$ indicate respiratory acidosis, and the normal HCO_3^- level means no compensation has occurred. A pH of 7.32, $PaCO_2$ of 60 mm Hg, and HCO_3^- level of 39 mEq/liter indicate compensated respiratory acidosis; a pH of 7.18, $PaCO_2$ of 34 mm Hg, and HCO_3^- level of 19 mEq/liter indicate uncompensated metabolic acidosis; a pH of 7.50, $PaCO_2$ of 25 mm Hg, and HCO_3^- level of 24 mEq/liter indicate uncompensated respiratory alkalosis.

44 Correct answer—**A**

The patient's body will attempt to compensate for respiratory acidosis by increasing ammonia ion formation and excretion. Potassium moving into the cell commonly accompanies respiratory alkalosis; it is not a compensatory mechanism for respiratory acidosis. A decreased respiratory rate and depth would worsen the patient's condition. Compensation causes the kidneys to decrease, not increase, HCO_3^- excretion.

45 Correct answer—**B**

During fluid resuscitation, a critical part of initial treatment, the burn patient should receive lactated Ringer's solution, which has an osmolality of 275 mOsm/kg of water and contains sodium, potassium, calcium, and chlorine. This isotonic solution helps maintain adequate intravascular volume after burn injuries, which cause large sodium and water losses from the intravascular compartment. Lactated Ringer's solution must be infused rapidly until the patient's hemodynamic status is stable; infusion is continued, usually at 4 ml/kg for each percent of the body surface area (BSA) burned, for the first 24 hours. Dextrose 5% in water is not given for fluid resuscitation because it does not correct electrolyte losses or increase the intravascular volume. Hypotonic saline solution would cause fluid to move into the cells, causing increased cellular destruction. Supplemental potassium replacement typically is not necessary because serum potassium levels usually are elevated from the existing cellular and muscle damage.

46 Correct answer—B

The patient's sex and past medical history would not influence immediate fluid resuscitation. The depth and BSA percentage of burns is the most crucial information for determining the patient's fluid requirements; the "Rule of Nines" helps in calculating these requirements. Hemoconcentration (reflected by increased hematocrit and hemoglobin values), oliguria, and increased urine specific gravity, which indicate a need for fluid, are common in the early stages of burn injuries; they result from intravascular depletion as body fluids shift into the intracellular and interstitial compartments. The nurse must carefully monitor urine output and specific gravity to assess for impending renal failure.

47 Correct answer—B

Plasma-to-interstitial fluid shift usually occurs during the intial stage of a burn injury; this causes leakage through the capillaries, resulting in edema. Because of cellular trauma, potassium is released into the extracellular space, causing hyperkalemia. After the initial stage, which usually lasts approximately 36 hours, the body starts to shift fluid back into the intravascular space, predisposing the patient to circulatory overload; at the same time, large amounts of potassium are excreted in the urine because of the increased intravascular volume. Aldosterone, which reabsorbs sodium and excretes potassium, is released in large quantities in response to dilutional hyponatremia, which develops as intracellular and interstitial fluid shift back into the intravascular compartment.

48 Correct answer—C

A decreased serum sodium level usually indicates dilutional hyponatremia, or water excess; the patient's water intake should be restricted to allow the kidneys to excrete the excess water. The other laboratory values do not reflect changes in water balance.

49 Correct answer—A

Hyperosmolality, not hypo-osmolality, occurs in the patient with diabetic ketoacidosis (DKA) because of increased serum glucose. When the serum glucose exceeds the tubular reabsorption capacity, glycosuria occurs, acting as an osmotic diuretic. Circulatory insufficiency follows; total fluid loss may equal 8 to 10 liters, resulting in increased hyperosmolality and severe dehydration. Excessive ketone production leads to metabolic acidosis, which causes potassium to move from the cells into the intravascular space. Although the total amount of potassium in the patient's body is low, serum potassium levels are elevated because of this shift. The body attempts to compensate for metabolic acidosis with hyperventilation, resulting in hypocapnia.

50 Correct answer—A

Isotonic saline solution is the most commonly used I.V. solution in the initial treatment of DKA. The patient with DKA usually has severe intravascular depletion and cellular dehydration; infusing isotonic saline solution promotes intravascular rehydration and stabilizes hemodynamic status. Once the circulatory system is stable but the cells are still dehydrated, body fluid repletion is achieved with a hypotonic solution, such as half-normal saline solution. After fluid therapy and insulin administration begin, the nurse must carefully monitor serum electrolyte and glucose levels. When the serum glucose level falls to 250 to 300 mg/dl, insulin is discontinued and fluid therapy changes to a hypertonic solution containing glucose, such as dextrose 5% in normal saline solution, to prevent the development of hypoglycemia, hypokalemia, and cerebral edema.

51 Correct answer—A

Lactulose (Chronulac) is used in patients with cirrhosis to decrease the ammonia level in the bloodstream; lactulose enemas are not used to treat hyperkalemia. When the serum potassium level exceeds 6.5 mEq/liter or electrocardiogram changes indicate severe hyperkalemia, the physician may order administration of glucose and insulin or sodium bicarbonate I.V. to temporarily shift potassium into the cells. Calcium chloride or calcium gluconate may be given I.V. to stimulate cardiac contractility. The physician also may order administration of sodium polystyrene sulfonate (Kayexalate) in sorbitol to promote potassium excretion from the body and reverse hyperkalemia.

52 Correct answer—A

Hyperkalemia commonly causes oliguria; mental status changes, such as apathy and confusion; GI changes, such as diarrhea and abdominal cramping; and neuromuscular changes, such as flaccid paralysis and numbness of the extremities. Tetany and bradypnea are signs of hypokalemia. Hyperactive bowel sounds and polyuria are not associated with hyperkalemia.

53 Correct answer—D

Metabolic acidosis typically results in elevated serum potassium levels; the excess hydrogen ions in the serum shift into the cells, causing potassium to shift from the cells into the serum. Hyperkalemia is not commonly associated with the other choices.

54 Correct answer—B

Hypophosphatemia is most commonly caused by chronic alcoholism; the alcoholic patient's nutrition typically is poor, causing an inadequate phosphate intake. Other causes include malabsorption problems, starvation, and total parenteral nutrition. Acute and chronic renal failure cause hyperphosphatemia; failing kidneys cannot excrete phosphates. Alkalosis accelerates phosphate passage from the serum into cells, but this rarely occurs.

55 Correct answer—B

Because phosphate and calcium have an inverse relationship, the calcium level is high when the phosphate level is low; thus, the clinical manifestations of hypercalcemia and hypophosphatemia are the same (manifestations include mental confusion, muscle weakness, anorexia, nausea, and impaired reflexes). Numbness around the mouth, carpopedal spasm, and muscle twitching and cramping are signs of hyperphosphatemia and hypocalcemia.

56 Correct answer—A

Initial treatment for hypophosphatemia should include the administration of potassium phosphate (Neutra-Phos-K) capsules diluted in water. The physician may order sodium phosphate or potassium phosphate I.V. if hypophosphatemia is severe. Acetazolamide (Diamox) and aluminum hydroxide (Amphojel) are not given because they would further decrease the serum phosphate level. Vitamin replacement would not be part of the patient's initial therapy because it would not eliminate low phosphate levels; phosphate is a mineral, not a vitamin.

CHAPTER 6

Musculoskeletal and Integumentary Systems

Questions

1 Which assessment finding indicates carbunculosis?

A. Extensive erythema and local tenderness
B. A painful, hard, red nodule surrounding a hair follicle
C. An extremely painful, hard, red nodule surrounding several hair follicles
D. Macular erythema with oozing vesicles

2 Which statement about skin cancer is *not* correct?

A. Skin cancer is most common in fair-complexioned whites
B. Skin cancer is directly related to the amount and intensity of electromagnetic radiation exposure
C. Skin cancer is more common in women than men
D. Skin cancer is more common in patients undergoing immunosuppressive therapy

---

SITUATION

Ms. B., a 30-year-old model, sustains an open fracture of her left wrist while roller skating.

Questions 3 to 5 refer to this situation.

3 Ms. B.'s fracture will be reduced and immobilized in the emergency department (ED) with a cast. Which nursing action is *not* indicated before the cast is applied?

A. Cleaning the wound with an antiseptic as ordered
B. Shaving the hair from the forearm
C. Drying the arm thoroughly
D. Gathering a container of water, plaster of Paris, and sheet wadding

4 Which assessment finding should the nurse report immediately to the physician after Ms. B.'s cast is applied?

A. Slight edema of the fingers
B. Warm, mobile fingers
C. Bright red drainage on the cast
D. Complaints of pain when the wrist is dependent

5 While caring for Ms. B. for the first 48 hours after her cast is applied, the nurse should:

A. Handle the cast with the palms of her hands
B. Keep the cast covered to speed its drying
C. Perform neurologic assessments every 8 hours
D. Position the cast on a hard surface

SITUATION

Mrs. C., age 78, is admitted to the surgical unit after a minor fall at home causes a right femoral neck (hip) fracture. She is placed in Buck's extension traction with a 5-lb weight and scheduled for surgery the following morning.

Questions 6 to 11 refer to this situation.

6 Initial assessment of Mrs. C. would most likely reveal:

A. Internal rotation and abduction of the right leg, which is shorter than the left leg
B. Lateral rotation and adduction of the right leg, which is shorter than the left leg
C. Heat and redness over the fracture site
D. Fever, chills, and an elevated white blood cell (WBC) count

7 When providing care for Mrs. C., the nurse should initially be concerned with:

A. Complications caused by immobility
B. Aseptic necrosis of the femoral head
C. Malposition of the femoral head
D. Shock and hemorrhage

8 Which statement is *not* true of Buck's extension traction?

A. It temporarily immobilizes the fracture
B. It prevents or decreases deformities
C. It reduces muscle spasms
D. It applies force to more than one bone

9 Which patient activity is contraindicated while Mrs. C. is in Buck's extension traction?

A. Using a fracture bedpan
B. Watching television in the high-Fowler's position
C. Performing isometric exercises with the affected leg
D. Using a trapeze to change position

10 Because Mrs. C. is immobile, she is assigned a nursing diagnosis of *Potential constipation due to limited mobility.* Which measure would be *least* effective for this diagnosis?

A. Forcing fluids (3,000 ml or more daily)
B. Ordering prune juice daily
C. Encouraging the patient to eat foods high in fiber
D. Changing the patient's position every 2 hours

11 After the physician performs a total hip replacement, the nurse should turn Mrs. C.:

A. On her affected side
B. On her unaffected side
C. With her legs crossed to prevent dislocation of the prosthesis
D. On her affected side with an abductor pillow under her hip

---

SITUATION

Mr. L., a 52-year-old lawyer, comes to the primary care clinic with redness, tenderness, and swelling of the metatarsophalangeal area of his left great toe. The physician diagnoses acute gout.

Questions 12 to 15 refer to this situation.

12 Gout is a disease involving abnormal purine metabolism, which results in increased serum levels of:

A. Lactic acid
B. Uric acid
C. Ascorbic acid
D. Pyruvic acid

13 Nursing care for Mr. L. during an acute gout attack probably would include:

A. Active range-of-motion (ROM) exercises of the affected extremity

B. Increased physical activity

C. Bed rest and elevation of the affected foot

D. Elevation of the affected foot, wrapped in an elastic bandage

14 Which medication is considered the drug of choice for treating gout?

A. Colchicine (Colsalide)

B. Allopurinol (Zyloprim)

C. Probenecid (Benemid)

D. Indomethacin (Indocin)

15 Before Mr. L. is discharged, the nurse should emphasize to him the importance of maintaining:

A. A diet rich in high-purine foods, such as sardines and organ meats

B. A regular exercise program

C. A fluid intake of 3,000 ml or more daily

D. Acidic urine

SITUATION

Mrs. M., age 70, visits the primary care clinic with complaints of an aching pain in her left hip. The physician diagnoses osteoarthritis of the left hip.

Questions 16 and 17 refer to this situation.

16 Expected findings during the nursing assessment would include:

A. Joint pain that increases with activity

B. Morning stiffness lasting several hours

C. Periarticular osteoporosis

D. Pannus formation

17 Before discharge, the nurse should give Mrs. M. all of the following instructions *except:*

A. "Sit down as much as possible"
B. "Stand and walk erect using good posture"
C. "Wear comfortable, supportive shoes"
D. "Take rest periods while exercising"

SITUATION

Mrs. F., a 46-year-old homemaker, is admitted to the hospital with a diagnosis of rheumatoid arthritis.

Questions 18 to 21 refer to this situation.

18 Which assessment finding should the nurse expect in Mrs. F.?

A. An asymmetrical pattern of affected joints
B. A positive rheumatoid factor titer
C. The presence of Heberden's nodes
D. A positive antinuclear antibody titer

19 Which type of medication is most commonly used to treat rheumatoid arthritis?

A. Glucocorticoids
B. Nonsteroidal anti-inflammatory drugs (NSAIDs)
C. Antimalarial drugs
D. Gold salts

20 Before discharge, the nurse tells Mrs. F. that she should pace her activities. An example of pacing activities would be:

A. Doing all her household chores in the morning and resting in the afternoon
B. Taking a nap before going shopping
C. Working hard on days her joints do not hurt and resting on days her joints are inflamed
D. Hiring a helper to do the housework

21 Which type of exercise should the nurse recommend to Mrs. F.?

A. Jogging
B. Swimming
C. Bicycling
D. Skating

22 Which diagnostic test result would help confirm Mr. J.'s diagnosis of ankylosing spondylitis?

A. The presence of rheumatoid factor
B. An elevated erythrocyte sedimentation rate
C. The presence of human leukocyte antigen B27
D. An elevated WBC count

23 Which assessment finding is *not* a common clinical manifestation of ankylosing spondylitis?

A. Flexion adduction deformities of the hips
B. Swollen joints in the knees and shoulders
C. Progressive diaphragmatic breathing
D. Arthralgia remission

SITUATION

Mrs. B., a 45-year-old secretary, visits the medical clinic with complaints of pain in her right hand and wrist. Nursing assessment reveals edematous fingers with numbness and paresthesia of the right hand and wrist. The physician suspects carpal tunnel syndrome.

Questions 24 to 27 refer to this situation.

24 Which nerve is compressed in carpal tunnel syndrome?

A. Median
B. Brachial plexus
C. Radial
D. Posterial tibial

25 Which assessment finding helps confirm the diagnosis of carpal tunnel syndrome?

A. Positive Homans' sign
B. Tinnitus
C. Positive Tinel's sign
D. Raynaud's phenomenon

26 The physician operates on Mrs. B.'s right wrist to relieve the nerve compression. The most important aspect of postoperative nursing assessment for Mrs. B. is:

A. Urinary and bowel function
B. Circulation to the right hand
C. Level of consciousness
D. Pain tolerance

27 During the early postoperative period, the nurse should teach Mrs. B. to:

A. Keep both arms elevated and immobile
B. Use her right hand as much as possible
C. Perform active ROM exercises with her right arm and wrist
D. Periodically make a fist with her right hand

SITUATION

Mr. B., age 28, sustained injuries during a motor vehicle accident resulting in an amputation of his right leg below the knee. He is to be fitted with a prosthesis.

Questions 28 and 29 refer to this situation.

28 Mr. B. experiences a burning sensation where his right foot used to be. What causes this phantom sensation?

A. The patient's imagination
B. Infection at the suture line of the amputated limb
C. Previous sensations from the area, which have been imprinted on the brain and remain even after the leg has been removed
D. Referred pain from the left foot

29 Which measure should *not* be part of Mr. B.'s stump care after the suture line has healed completely?

A. Daily cleaning of the stump with a nondeodorant soap
B. Rinsing the stump well with warm water
C. Air-drying the stump for at least 30 minutes
D. Briskly rubbing the stump dry with a clean towel

SITUATION

Mrs. G., age 65, has had unremitting pain in both knees for 7 years because of osteoarthritis. The physician has scheduled a total replace-

ment of her left knee.

Questions 30 to 32 refer to this situation.

30 To prevent preoperative thrombophlebitis, the nurse should instruct Mrs. G. on:

A. Active flexion of the foot
B. Isotonic exercises for the knees
C. Straight leg raising every 2 hours
D. Wearing antiembolism stockings while ambulating

31 Mrs. G.'s leg is connected to a continuous passive motion device before she is taken from the operating room after the procedure. The primary purpose of this device is to:

A. Promote early weight bearing
B. Increase circulation and movement
C. Prevent foot drop
D. Support and elevate the leg

32 The physician schedules Mrs. G. for postoperative bedside physical therapy. Which nursing diagnosis should *not* be included in her care plan?

A. Pain related to the surgical procedure
B. Potential for impaired skin integrity related to decreased mobility
C. Knowledge deficit related to surgical procedure
D. Impaired physical mobility related to musculoskeletal impairment

SITUATION

Mr. R., a 36-year-old firefighter, has experienced burns over his anterior face, neck, chest, and arms while fighting an explosive fire in an oil refinery. He is brought to the ED.

Questions 33 to 36 refer to this situation.

33 Which assessment finding indicates a partial-thickness burn?

A. Hair follicles that are easily pulled out
B. Large, moist vesicles
C. Lack of skin blanching with pressure
D. Little or no pain in the burned area

34 Mr. R. is scheduled for debridement and wound cleaning. The physician orders a small dose of meperidine (Demerol) before the procedure. Which route of administration would be most appropriate?

A. I.V.
B. I.M.
C. Subcutaneous
D. Intradermal

35 Which topical antibacterial agent commonly used on burns penetrates the eschar?

A. Silver sulfadiazine (Silvadene)
B. Mafenide acetate (Sulfamylon)
C. 0.5% silver nitrate solution
D. 10% povidone-iodine (Betadine) solution

36 The physician decides to cover Mr. R.'s facial wounds with an allograft. Which statement best describes an allograft?

A. Tissue taken from an animal
B. Tissue taken from another area of the patient's body
C. Tissue taken from a person other than the patient
D. Tissue taken from amniotic membrane

SITUATION

Mrs. S., age 36, is admitted to the allergy clinic with urticaria and angioedema that developed after eating at a friend's dinner party.

Questions 37 and 38 refer to this situation.

37 The physician orders diphenhydramine (Benadryl). Which type of effect does this drug have on allergic reactions?

A. Antipyretic
B. Antiemetic
C. Antihistamine
D. Antivertigo

38 Mrs. S. is also given hydrocortisone (Deltacort) ointment to apply to the affected areas. The best method for applying this ointment is:

A. Gently smoothing a small amount of medication on the affected area
B. Rubbing the medication firmly into the skin
C. Patting the medication onto the skin with a clean gauze pad
D. Placing the ointment on gauze and taping it over the affected area

SITUATION

Mr. G., age 33, is admitted to the medical unit with severe psoriasis. He has severe pain and fissures in his elbows and knees. Mr. G. states that his condition has not responded to creams recommended by his physician.

Questions 39 to 43 refer to this situation.

39 Which assessment finding is most characteristic of psoriasis?

A. White or yellowish macules and papules on the scalp
B. Elevated plaques of skin with silvery scales
C. Multiple blisters with encrustation
D. Hair loss, primarily on the scalp

40 Which factor does *not* exacerbate psoriasis?

A. Poor personal hygiene
B. Stress
C. Infection
D. Surgical incisions

41 Treatment of psoriasis is aimed at reducing the rapid epidermal proliferation and associated inflammation. Which intervention should the nurse expect in Mr. G.'s treatment?

A. Topical application of steroids
B. Methotrexate sodium (Mexate) by I.V. push
C. Soaks with Burow's solution
D. Topical diphenhydramine

42 Which laboratory test results should the nurse review to detect drug toxicity?

A. Serum glucose level
B. Serum triglyceride level
C. Liver function test results
D. Blood urea nitrogen level

43 The nurse should cover all of the following topics with Mr. G. during discharge teaching *except:*

A. The need to continue treatment with prescribed creams and ointments and to avoid precipitating factors
B. Referral to the National Psoriasis Foundation
C. The need to refrain from pulling at lesions
D. Instructions to take frequent hot baths to remove scales

SITUATION

Mrs. D., a 66-year-old patient immobilized for a fractured hip, develops a pressure ulcer on the sacrum. The physician orders application of a proteolytic enzyme ointment with a wet dressing followed by a dry sterile dressing each shift, as well as systemic antibiotic therapy for the infection.

Questions 44 and 45 refer to this situation.

44 Proteolytic enzyme ointment is given to:

A. Liberate oxygen in the wound
B. Absorb purulent exudate from the wound
C. Dissolve inaccessible necrotic tissue
D. Cause moisture-reactive particles to create a soft gel over the wound

45 Before Mrs. D.'s systemic antibiotic therapy begins, the nurse should:

A. Wash the wound with normal saline solution and hydrogen peroxide
B. Determine the patient's body weight and calculate the drug dosage
C. Remove eschar to allow the cells to breathe
D. Take a drainage specimen for culture and sensitivity

SITUATION

While caring for Mr. H., age 72, the nurse notices vesicles on one side of his chest that were not present the previous day. Further assessment reveals some encrustation. The patient appears lethargic, has a low-grade temperature, and complains of pain over the area. The physician suspects herpes zoster.

Questions 46 to 49 refer to this situation.

---

46 Which assessment finding helps confirm the diagnosis of herpes zoster?

A. Encrustation of the vesicles
B. Grouping of the vesicles on one side of the chest
C. Pain associated with the vesicles
D. A low-grade fever

47 Individuals who develop herpes zoster commonly have a history of:

A. Streptococcal laryngitis (strep throat)
B. Contact with an infected pet
C. Sharing clothing with a roommate
D. Exposure to chicken pox

48 Which drug should the physician order for Mr. H. to render the virus ineffective?

A. Indomethacin (Indocin)
B. Cyanocobalamin (vitamin B$_{12}$)
C. Acyclovir sodium (Zovirax)
D. Methylprednisolone sodium succinate (Solu-Medrol)

49 The most effective intervention in preventing the transmission of herpes zoster is:

A. Thorough hand washing and the use of gloves
B. Respiratory isolation
C. Limited sexual contact
D. Reverse isolation

SITUATION

Mr. S., a 51-year-old bank vice-president, consults a physician because a preexisting nevus (mole) on his forearm has become itchy and changed in size and color. Mr. S. has fair skin, blue eyes, and light hair; his sun exposure usually is intermittent but intense on weekends. The physician suspects malignant melanoma.

Questions 50 and 51 refer to this situation.

50 Which assessment finding does *not* indicate malignant melanoma?

A. Asymmetry and border irregularity
B. Nonuniform color
C. Positive computed tomography scan
D. Diameter greater than 6 mm

51 Which health history finding would be considered a risk factor for the development of malignant melanoma?

A. Changes in bowel movement pattern
B. Overexposure to sunlight and X-rays
C. History of nausea, vomiting, and alopecia
D. Family history of lung cancer

An excision biopsy of Mr. S.'s nevus confirms the diagnosis; the tumor is classified as superficial spreading melanoma at stage II. The physician performs a wide excision of the tumor and orders dacarbazine (DTIC-Dome) chemotherapy.

Questions 52 and 53 continue the situation.

52 Which adverse effects should the nurse expect in Mr. S. following administration of dacarbazine?

A. Flulike symptoms
B. Red urine
C. Cardiotoxicity
D. Fluid retention

53 Before discharge, the nurse should instruct Mr. S. to take all of the following measures *except:*

A. Having follow-up medical examinations
B. Protecting his skin from overexposure to the sun
C. Avoiding sun lamps and tanning parlors
D. Using baby oil to protect the skin when exposed to the sun

Answer sheet

A B C D	A B C D
1 ○ ○ ○ ○	31 ○ ○ ○ ○
2 ○ ○ ○ ○	32 ○ ○ ○ ○
3 ○ ○ ○ ○	33 ○ ○ ○ ○
4 ○ ○ ○ ○	34 ○ ○ ○ ○
5 ○ ○ ○ ○	35 ○ ○ ○ ○
6 ○ ○ ○ ○	36 ○ ○ ○ ○
7 ○ ○ ○ ○	37 ○ ○ ○ ○
8 ○ ○ ○ ○	38 ○ ○ ○ ○
9 ○ ○ ○ ○	39 ○ ○ ○ ○
10 ○ ○ ○ ○	40 ○ ○ ○ ○
11 ○ ○ ○ ○	41 ○ ○ ○ ○
12 ○ ○ ○ ○	42 ○ ○ ○ ○
13 ○ ○ ○ ○	43 ○ ○ ○ ○
14 ○ ○ ○ ○	44 ○ ○ ○ ○
15 ○ ○ ○ ○	45 ○ ○ ○ ○
16 ○ ○ ○ ○	46 ○ ○ ○ ○
17 ○ ○ ○ ○	47 ○ ○ ○ ○
18 ○ ○ ○ ○	48 ○ ○ ○ ○
19 ○ ○ ○ ○	49 ○ ○ ○ ○
20 ○ ○ ○ ○	50 ○ ○ ○ ○
21 ○ ○ ○ ○	51 ○ ○ ○ ○
22 ○ ○ ○ ○	52 ○ ○ ○ ○
23 ○ ○ ○ ○	53 ○ ○ ○ ○
24 ○ ○ ○ ○	
25 ○ ○ ○ ○	
26 ○ ○ ○ ○	
27 ○ ○ ○ ○	
28 ○ ○ ○ ○	
29 ○ ○ ○ ○	
30 ○ ○ ○ ○	

Answers and rationales

1 Correct answer—**C**

Clinical manifestations of carbunculosis include an extremely painful, hard, red nodule surrounding several hair follicles accompanied by fever and leukocytosis. Because the infection is not walled off, absorption of the infecting organism occurs, causing an elevated white blood cell (WBC) count, fever, and pain. A painful, hard, red nodule surrounding a single hair follicle is a furuncle or boil. Extensive erythema and local tenderness indicate cellulitis. Macular erythema with oozing vesicles is associated with impetigo.

2 Correct answer—**C**

Skin cancer, particularly squamous and basal cell cancers, is more common in men than women. Because it is more common in people who lack melanin, it is most common in fair-complexioned whites. Exposure to electromagnetic radiation has a direct carcinogenic effect; it interferes with cell-mediated immunity in the skin. Skin cancer is somewhat more common in immunosuppressed patients, such as those with renal transplants or on methotrexate therapy.

3 Correct answer—**B**

Shaving an open fracture site before applying a cast is not recommended because it may cause additional breaks in the skin, increasing the risk of infection. Nursing actions before applying a cast usually include washing the broken skin with an antiseptic as ordered and drying the affected limb thoroughly. (The cast for an open fracture typically has an opening to allow for treatment of the broken skin.) The nurse should gather all necessary materials—including a large container of water, plaster of Paris, and sheet wadding—so that the physician can apply the cast quickly, preventing further soft tissue damage.

4 Correct answer—**C**

Bright red drainage on a cast usually indicates active bleeding; the nurse should report this finding to the physician immediately. Some edema of the fingers is expected with this type of injury; elevating the arm should reduce the edema. If it persists or worsens with elevation, the nurse should call the physician. Warm, mobile fingers indicate adequate circulation and need not be reported. Leaving the patient's wrist dependent may cause pain and increased edema and should be avoided.

5 Correct answer—A

Until the cast is dry (typically 48 hours or more), the nurse should move the cast with the palms of her hands to avoid indenting it; indentations may cause pressure ulcers. A cast made of plaster of paris contains gypsum, which releases heat as it dries; covering the cast would increase this heat, possibly causing tissue damage. The nurse should perform neurologic assessment every 2 hours to reveal vascular impairment as well as previously undetected nerve damage. The nurse should not position the cast on a hard surface while it dries; this may cause pressure and indentation of the soft tissue underneath.

6 Correct answer—B

Lateral rotation of the affected leg is a classic sign of hip fracture; adduction and leg shortening also may be present, depending on the severity of the fracture. Abduction and internal rotation are rarely seen with hip fractures. Heat and redness over the fracture site, fever, chills, and an elevated WBC count are signs of infection and inflammation, which usually are not present during the initial stage of a fracture.

7 Correct answer—D

Because an elderly patient is at high risk for shock and hemorrhage after even a minor injury, the nurse should observe the patient closely for any change in vital signs. Complications caused by immobility, such as atelectasis, constipation, and skin breakdown, are not inital nursing concerns because the patient has not been immobilized for a long period. Aseptic necrosis of the femoral head results from the fracture and traumatic dislocation of the hip, and malposition of the femoral head probably is caused by the fracture as well; because surgical treatment of the fracture should prevent aseptic necrosis and correct malposition of the femoral head, these are not initial nursing concerns.

8 Correct answer—D

Buck's extension traction does not apply force to more than one bone; it is a type of skin traction that applies force in one direction. Buck's extension traction temporarily immobilizes the fracture, reduces muscle spasms, and prevents or decreases deformities. It typically is used until the physician performs internal fixation; it is used as a primary method of treatment only if the patient is too debilitated to undergo surgery.

9 Correct answer—B

Watching television in high-Fowler's position is contraindicated because it reduces the counterforce necessary to maintain proper bone alignment. A weight is used with traction to apply a force that immobilizes the fragmented ends and permits healing: with Buck's extension traction, a counterforce is necessary to maintain bone alignment and force. This counterforce is provided by the patient's body; therefore, the patient's position can alter the effectiveness of Buck's extension traction. If necessary, the counterforce may be increased by elevating the foot of the bed. Some orthopedic units permit the patient's head to be elevated 45 degrees at mealtime so she can eat more easily. By using a fracture bedpan, the patient may relieve herself without changing her position, maintaining the proper countercontraction. The patient needs some exercise of the affected leg to maintain muscle tone and prevent muscle atrophy; isometric exercises can be performed while immobile without misaligning the fractured bone. The trapeze allows the patient to move up in bed, preventing the complications caused by constant pressure on blood vessels and skin; using the trapeze also strengthens the patient's muscles and simplifies bed making.

10 Correct answer—D

The least effective intervention for potential constipation in this patient is changing position every 2 hours. Because the patient is in traction, only small changes in position are possible without disrupting bone healing; this will not prevent constipation. The other measures will help prevent constipation without disrupting the traction forces. Fluids soften fecal mass; prune juice helps stimulate peristalsis; and foods high in fiber increase bulk, also stimulating peristalsis.

11 Correct answer—B

The nurse should turn the patient on her unaffected side when the physician orders, usually several days after surgery. An abductor pillow or splint is placed between the patient's legs to prevent leg adduction and possible dislocation of the prosthesis. The patient with a hip prosthesis should not cross her legs for 3 to 4 months after surgery because this may cause dislocation.

12 Correct answer—B

Uric acid is the end product of purine metabolism; therefore, gout results in hyperuricemia. Excess uric acid crystals are deposited in joints and connective tissue, causing clinical manifestations of the diseases. Elevated serum lactic acid levels occur with liver disease, congestive heart failure, hemorrhage, and shock. Ascorbic acid, or vitamin C, levels do not affect purine metabolism. Elevated serum pyruvic acid levels are seen with diabetes, thiamine deficiency, and some infections.

13 Correct answer—C

For a patient in the acute phase of gout, the physician usually orders bed rest and elevation of the affected extremity to reduce edema and promote venous return. Because an acute episode of gout can cause severe pain and sensitivity, the patient may need a bed cradle to keep the bed linens off the affected foot. Range-of-motion exercises of the affected extremity, increased physical activity, and dressings or bandages on the affected foot would only increase the patient's pain.

14 Correct answer—A

Colchicine (Colsalide) is the drug of choice for treating gout because of its effective anti-inflammatory action; it appears to inhibit the migration of leukocytes into the inflamed area, decreasing the inflammatory response. Colchicine is most effective if given early in the course of the disease. The other choices typically are used to treat gout only after colchicine proves ineffective. Allopurinol (Zyloprim) reduces uric acid production. Probenecid (Benemid), a uricosuric agent, blocks the reabsorption and promotes the excretion of urates. Indomethacin (Indocin), a nonsteroidal anti-inflammatory drug (NSAID), is used to treat rheumatoid arthritis as well as gout.

15 Correct answer—C

A high fluid intake reduces the risk of urate precipitation in the kidney tubules of the patient with a history of gout. High-purine foods, such as sardines and organ meats, are not recommended for patients with a history of gout; they increase the risk of uric acid precipitation in the urinary system. A regular exercise program is a routine health promotion measure and does not have increased importance for a patient with gout. The patient's urine should be alkaline, not acidic, to prevent uric acid precipitation.

16 Correct answer—A

Joint pain increases with activity in osteoarthritis; it usually lessens with rest. Morning stiffness occurs with osteoarthritis but usually lasts 1 hour at most. Periarticular osteoporosis (reduction of bone mass around the joint cartilage) and pannus formation (overgrowth of inflammatory tissue over the surface of the joint cartilage outside the capsule) occur with rheumatoid arthritis, not osteoarthritis.

17 Correct answer—**A**

The nurse should not encourage the patient to sit because it may lead to flexion contractures and hip adduction. Good posture helps decrease excessive wear on weight-bearing joints. Supportive shoes provide less strain on weight-bearing joints and promote better posture. The patient should exercise, but she must remember to take rest periods to reduce joint stress.

18 Correct answer—**B**

Approximately 80% of patients with rheumatoid arthritis have a positive rheumatoid factor titer. A high titer on the latex fixation test, which makes up part of the rheumatoid factor titer, indicates severe disease. An asymmetrical pattern of affected joints and the presence of Heberden's nodes are characteristic of osteoarthritis, not rheumatoid arthritis. The patient with rheumatoid arthritis may have a positive antinuclear antibody titer, but this finding is not as common as a positive rheumatoid factor.

19 Correct answer—**B**

NSAIDs, such as aspirin, ibuprofen (Motrin), tolmetin (Tolectin), piroxicam (Feldene), and naproxen (Naprosyn), are most commonly used to treat rheumatoid arthritis because of their high effectiveness and minimal adverse patient reactions. Glucocorticoids, the antimalarial drug hydroxychloroquine sulfate (Plaquenil), and gold salts may be used to treat rheumatoid arthritis; however, these drugs are less commonly used because they are less effective and have more serious adverse effects than NSAIDs.

20 Correct answer—**B**

Taking a nap before going shopping is an example of pacing activities—balancing rest and physical activity to prevent fatigue and avoid overstraining the joints. Doing all the household chores in the morning and working hard when feeling well may exacerbate inflammation by overstraining the joints. Hiring a helper to do the housework is a way of reducing the amount of physical activity, not of pacing it.

21 Correct answer—**B**

Swimming is the best exercise for the patient with rheumatoid arthritis; the water supports the patient while she moves her joints, decreasing strain and the risk of injury from falls. Jogging, bicycling, and skating are not recommended because the motions involved increase the strain on the joints; also, the risk of injury from falls is increased with bicycling and skating.

22 Correct answer—C

The presence of human leukocyte antigen B27 would help confirm the diagnosis of ankylosing spondylitis; nearly 90% of patients with this disease have the antigen in their serum. The rheumatoid factor would not be present with ankylosing spondylitis unless it was caused by rheumatoid arthritis. An elevated erythrocyte sedimentation rate and WBC count accompany many disorders; these findings would not help confirm the diagnosis.

23 Correct answer—D

Arthralgia remission is a clinical manifestation of Reiter's syndrome, not ankylosing spondylitis. Ankylosing spondylitis is characterized by progressive inflammation of the spine and large joints (hip, shoulders, and knees), which leads to bone and cartilage deterioration. The pain from inflamed, swollen joints causes muscle spasms, producing flexion adduction deformities. Increased rounding and immobility of the spine reduces vital capacity, causing progressively limited chest motion and diaphragmatic breathing.

24 Correct answer—A

Carpal tunnel syndrome is an entrapment neuropathy caused by compression of the median nerve on the ventral surface of the wrist. Brachial nerve plexus compression may result from injuries of the shoulder and upper arm. Radial nerve compression occurs with trauma to the shoulder or elbow. Posterior tibial nerve compression may cause tarsal tunnel syndrome.

25 Correct answer—C

A positive Tinel's sign—a tingling sensation when the median nerve is tapped—indicates nerve irritability. A positive Homans' sign—pain in the calf when the foot is dorsiflexed—indicates thrombophlebitis or thrombosis. Tinnitus is a ringing heard in one or both ears, which indicates Ménière's disease. Raynaud's phenomenon refers to intermittent attacks of ischemia of the fingers and toes; it occurs with various diseases, including scleroderma, systemic lupus erythematosus, and Raynaud's disease.

26 Correct answer—B

Checking the circulation to the hand is the most important aspect of nursing assessment after surgery of the wrist or arm. The fingers should be warm and pink and should move freely; when the nurse applies pressure over the fingernails until they blanch, capillary refill should be within normal limits. Assessing the patient's urinary and bowel function and level of consciousness are basic nursing assessments after any surgical procedure. Pain tolerance is not commonly assessed after surgery.

27 Correct answer—D

Making a fist with the affected hand promotes flexibility and mobility, as well as circulation to the hand. Only the right arm and wrist should be kept elevated to promote venous return and reduce postoperative swelling; the right wrist should be kept immobile with a splint to maintain support and prevent trauma to the surgical site. The patient's care should include active and passive ROM exercises for all extremities except the right arm and wrist.

28 Correct answer—C

Phantom sensation is the result of the brain imprinting sensations and movements of the body before amputation; although the leg has been amputated, the brain continues to send impulses to the area and interprets certain impulses as originating in that area. Because these sensations are caused by interpretation of nerve impulses in the brain, they cannot be called imaginary. Infection of the suture line would probably not cause a burning sensation. Pain may be referred from one area of the body to another but not from one extremity to the other, even when both are present.

29 Correct answer—D

Briskly rubbing the stump could damage tissue subject to wear and stress under the prosthesis. Daily cleaning of the stump is necessary to prevent infection. Nondeodorant soap is used to prevent irritation. Rinsing well with warm water helps prevent the buildup of soapy films that may cause irritation and skin breakdown. Air drying is necessary to prevent skin maceration; it may be done before bedtime to permit complete overnight drying of the stump.

30 Correct answer—A

Before a total knee replacement, Mrs. G. should receive instructions about active flexion of the foot. This action increases skeletal muscle contraction and increases venous return, which helps prevent thrombophlebitis. Isotonic exercise involves muscle contraction without resistance, which shortens muscles without increasing muscle tone or strength; this type of exercise would be ineffective at preventing thrombophlebitis, and the patient might not be able to perform isotonic knee exercises because of the pain in her knees. Straight leg raising would be more beneficial in strengthening muscles than preventing thrombophlebitis. To prevent thrombophlebitis, the patient should wear antiembolism stockings at all times, not just when she ambulates.

31 Correct answer—B

The primary purpose of the continuous passive motion (CPM) device is to increase circulation and movement by providing CPM to the leg. The physician determines the degree of extension and flexion that the motorized, splintlike device will provide as well as the period it will operate. The same device is used after discharge. It does not prevent foot drop or promote early weight bearing. Pillows usually are used to elevate and support the leg.

32 Correct answer—C

Knowledge deficit related to surgical procedure may be appropriate before surgery but not afterward. *Potential for impaired skin integrity* may result from the surgical incision or immobility after the procedure; it may lead to tissue breakdown. The procedure may cause postoperative pain. Musculoskeletal impairment from joint disease is the reason for surgery, and the procedure will limit the patient's mobility for a time.

33 Correct answer—B

By definition, a partial-thickness (second-degree) burn destroys the epidermis and typically causes the formation of moist vesicles, a pink or mottled-red skin appearance that blanches under pressure, and pain in the burned area. Because the epidermal cells lining the hair follicles are not destroyed, the hair follicles are not easily pulled out.

34 Correct answer—A

The I.V. route ensures that the prescribed dose reaches the central nervous system. The I.M., subcutaneous, and intradermal routes are not recommended because of poor absorption (caused by decreased circulation and fluid shift to the extravascular space), eschar formation, and damaged tissue present with burns. If the I.V. route is not used, the patient may inadvertently receive inadequate medication for achieving pain control or too much medication, which may lead to respiratory depression.

35 Correct answer—B

Mafenide acetate (Sulfamylon) will penetrate tissue and burn eschar. It is most effective against *Pseudomonas aeruginosa*. Unfortunately, its application may be painful; also, because mafenide acetate and its metabolites are strong carbonic anhydrase inhibitors, metabolic acidosis may develop. Silver nitrate is used for its antibacterial action against fungal organisms, but it does not penetrate eschar as well as mafenide acetate. Silver sulfadiazine (Silvadene) is applied only to debrided areas because it does not penetrate eschar. Povidone-iodine (Betadine) solution, an antiseptic agent, does not penetrate eschar and irritates damaged tissue; it should not be applied to burns except for surface cleaning.

36 Correct answer—C

An allograft, or homograft, is taken from a person other than the patient. Exposed burn tissue must be protected because it is extremely vulnerable to infection. Grafting protects the tissue and helps control fluid loss and body temperature. Tissue taken from an animal is called a xenograft or heterograft; pigskin is a commonly used xenograft. Tissue taken from the patient's body is called an autograft. In severely burned patients, donor sites for autografts may be severely limited; the physician may use tissue from another person to cover the wound until autografting is possible. Tissue taken from amniotic membrane is a particular type of allograft; it typically is used as a temporary biological dressing rather than as a permanent graft material.

37 Correct answer—C

Diphenhydramine (Benadryl) has an antihistamine effect; it competes with H_1 receptor sites on effector cells, blocking histamine release. This drug has no effect on the body's temperature regulating center. It does have an antiemetic effect; however, this effect does not alleviate allergic reaction symptoms. Diphenhydramine does not have an antivertigo effect.

38 Correct answer—A

The best method for applying ointment is gently smoothing a small amount of medication on the affected area, which ensures even distribution and prevents skin irritation. Rubbing the skin can cause irritation. Patting and the use of a rough material, such as gauze, may also cause irritation; additionally, occlusive dressings are rarely used with ointments.

39 Correct answer—**B**

Elevated plaques of skin with silvery scales is the most common clinical manifestation of psoriasis; the disease causes chronic epidermal cell proliferation, producing lesions that resemble thick silvery scales. These lesions are found on bony prominences as well as the trunk and scalp. Multiple blisters with encrustation is not common with psoriasis. White or yellowish macules and papules and hair loss on the scalp are characteristic of alopecia; they are not associated with psoriasis.

40 Correct answer—**A**

Psoriasis is not exacerbated by poor personal hygiene. Exacerbations appear to be linked to certain genetic and environmental factors, such as stress, infection, and surgical incisions; an alteration in the immune system causing rapid proliferation may also be involved.

41 Correct answer—**B**

Methotrexate sodium (Mexate) I.V. is the usual treatment for severe psoriasis that does not respond to creams and topical ointments; this antimetabolite drug inhibits the synthesis of deoxyribonucleic acid (DNA) in epidermal cells. Steroids cause a local decrease in epidermal cell activity, but they are not effective or fast enough to treat severe psoriasis. Burow's solution, which has an astringent effect, should not be used to treat this patient because it would cause additional dryness of the skin. Diphenhydramine provides temporary relief from itching, but it does not treat the epidermal proliferation and inflammation.

42 Correct answer—**C**

To assess the patient for toxicity to methotrexate sodium, the nurse should review liver function test results, such as the serum aspartate aminotransferase (formerly serum glutamic-oxaloacetic transaminase) level, serum alanine aminotransferase (formerly serum glutamic-pyruvic transaminase) level, and liver biopsy findings. The drug is administered in low doses because it is toxic to the liver. The drug also has a depressant effect on the bone marrow; therefore, the patient should have complete blood counts performed on a regular basis. Methotrexate sodium can elevate the serum glucose level, but this is not considered a toxic effect. Because the serum triglyceride level can be altered by food intake as well as liver dysfunction, it is not a good indicator of drug toxicity. Blood urea nitrogen level abnormalities indicate kidney, not liver, malfunction.

43 Correct answer—D

The nurse should not instruct the patient to take hot baths to remove scaling; hot water dries the skin and may worsen the condition. The nurse should emphasize to the patient the importance of continuing treatment and avoiding factors that precipitate and exacerbate the condition. Pulling at lesions should be discouraged because it may break the skin, possibly resulting in infection. The nurse should provide information about resource groups, such as the National Psoriasis Foundation.

44 Correct answer—C

Proteolytic enzymes, such as fibrinolysin and desoxyribonuclease (Elase) and sutilains (Travase), dissolve or digest necrotic tissue in wounds. Their action is enhanced by a moist environment; therefore, gauze wet with normal saline solution is applied after the ointment. Pulling off the wet dressing to apply the dry one helps debride the wound by removing dead tissue. Hydrogen peroxide liberates oxygen from wounds. Hydrophilic agents, such as Mesalt and Bard absorption agents, absorb purulent exudate. Such dressings as Op-Site, Duoderm, and Tegaderm allow moisture-reactive particles to create a soft gel over the wound.

45 Correct answer—D

Before systemic antibiotic therapy for an infected pressure ulcer begins, the nurse should take a drainage specimen for culture and sensitivity to identify the microorganisms present and determine which drug would be most effective against them; this prevents adverse effects from the indiscriminate use of antibiotics, a particular problem in an elderly patient. Washing the wound with normal saline solution and hydrogen peroxide may remove drainage and clean the ulcer, but this would not affect the infection or antibiotic therapy. The nurse should determine the patient's body weight, but the physician uses this information to calculate the drug dosage. The nurse should not remove eschar because this may lead to scarring.

46 Correct answer—B

Unilateral lesions that do not cross the midline help confirm a diagnosis of herpes zoster; with this disease, vesicles follow the pathway of the nerves from the posterior ganglia, involving the cranial, cervical, thoracic, lumbar, and sacral nerves. Encrustation of vesicles is common with dermatologic problems. Pain occurs with many diseases besides herpes zoster. A low-grade fever is a bodily reaction to bacterial growth, which is common with many diseases.

47 Correct answer—D

Herpes zoster is caused by certain DNA viruses that are also responsible for chicken pox; some authorities believe that herpes zoster results from reactivation of a latent case of chicken pox, in which the individual has become only partly immune. Exposure to and subsequent infection with chicken pox typically renders an individual immune to recurrence of chicken pox but not necessarily to herpes, which can recur repeatedly. It also occurs more frequently with patients whose immune system is depressed, such as those with lymphomas or leukemia. A history of strep throat is associated with rheumatic fever, not herpes zoster. Contact with infected pets may lead to the development of ringworm (tinea). Sharing clothing with someone may lead to scabies (mites) if the other person is infected.

48 Correct answer—C

The physician should order acyclovir sodium (Zovirax) to render the virus ineffective; this antiviral drug halts disease progression by inhibiting the virus DNA synthesis. Indomethacin (Indocin) is a nonsteroidal anti-inflammatory drug with an analgesic effect; it would not render the virus ineffective. Neurotropic vitamins, such as B_{12}, are sometimes recommended; however, research has not proven their therapeutic effectiveness. Methylprednisolone sodium succinate (Solu-Medrol), a steroid that causes immunosuppression, is contraindicated in systemic infections because it may lead to superinfection.

49 Correct answer—A

The most effective intervention to prevent herpes zoster transmission is thorough hand washing and the use of gloves. Respiratory isolation is not effective because the virus is spread by contact with the fluid-filled vesicles, not by droplets in the air. Reverse isolation protects an immunosuppressed patient from being infected by staff members; it is inappropriate for this situation. Herpes genitalis, not herpes zoster, is transmitted by sexual contact; limited sexual contact would not prevent herpes zoster transmission.

50 Correct answer—C

Computed tomography is not used to diagnose malignant melanoma. A tissue sample must be examined microscopically to confirm the diagnosis and determine the tumor's thickness. Asymmetry, border irregularity, color nonuniformity, and diameter greater than 6 mm (called the ABCD rule) indicate malignant melanoma.

51 Correct answer—**B**

Risk factors for the development of malignant melanoma include overexposure to sunlight, repeated medical and industrial X-ray exposure, scarring from disease or burns, and occupational exposure to such compounds as coal and arsenic. Changes in bowel movement pattern, a history of nausea, vomiting, and alopecia, and a family history of lung cancer are not risk factors for the development of malignant melanoma.

52 Correct answer—**A**

Dacarbazine (DTIC-Dome) causes flulike symptoms of nausea, vomiting, and diarrhea as well as anaphylaxis and pain on administration; delayed toxicity of the drug causes bone marrow depression, ototoxicity, hemolysis, hypomagnesemia, peripheral neuropathy, hypocalcemia, and hypokalemia. Red urine, cardiotoxicity, and fluid retention are not adverse effects of dacarbazine.

53 Correct answer—**D**

Baby oil offers no protection from exposure to the sun. When exposure is unavoidable, dermatologists recommend sunscreens with a protection factor of 15 and above. Follow-up medical examinations are recommended to check for recurrence. Minimizing sun exposure (especially between 10 a.m. and 3 p.m., when sun rays are strongest), covering the skin with clothing, wearing wide-brimmed hats to reduce face and neck exposure, and avoiding sun lamps and tanning parlors are also recommended because ultraviolet rays increase the risk of developing malignant melanoma.

CHAPTER 7

Endocrine and Reproductive Systems

Questions

1 Which complication of diabetes mellitus is indicated by Kussmaul's respirations?

A. Hyperosmolar nonketotic syndrome
B. Diabetic ketoacidosis
C. Gastroparesis
D. Glomerulosclerosis

2 Which medication is *not* an oral hypoglycemic agent?

A. Chlorpropamide (Diabinese)
B. Glipizide (Glucotrol)
C. Diazoxide (Hyperstat)
D. Tolbutamide (Orinase)

3 When caring for Mrs. V., a diabetic patient starting prednisone (Deltasone) therapy for severe arthritis, the nurse should expect:

A. Improved diabetes control
B. Worsened diabetes control
C. No effect on diabetes control
D. Frequent hypoglycemic reactions

4 Which is the most important self-care measure for an obese adult with newly diagnosed Type II (non-insulin-dependent) diabetes?

A. Monitoring blood glucose levels daily
B. Avoiding sugar-containing foods completely
C. Adhering strictly to the American Diabetes Association exchange diet
D. Reducing body weight

5 What is the most likely cause of consistent early-morning fasting hyperglycemia in a stable diabetic patient who takes one injection of isophane insulin suspension (NPH) each morning and has normal blood glucose levels throughout the remainder of the day?

A. Excessive evening snacks
B. Insufficient overnight insulin
C. The dawn phenomenon
D. Rebound hyperglycemia

6 Which nursing action should the nurse consider first when planning care for Mr. G., a 56-year-old patient with a 5-year history of poorly controlled diabetes?

A. Exploring with the patient his reasons for noncompliance
B. Arranging a family conference to discuss the patient's noncompliance
C. Teaching the patient about the complications associated with poorly controlled diabetes
D. Assessing the patient's knowledge and skill in diabetes management

7 A diabetic patient who takes NPH each morning experiences a hypoglycemic reaction at 2 a.m.; his blood glucose level is 50 mg/dl by the fingerstick method. The nurse gives him 6 oz of orange juice; at 6 a.m., his blood glucose level is 325 mg/dl. This elevation in blood glucose is probably caused by:

A. Excessive orange juice
B. Insufficient insulin
C. Rebound hyperglycemia
D. The dawn phenomenon

8 Which diabetes patient has the greatest need of a meticulous foot care regimen?

A. One with newly diagnosed diabetes
B. One with a 10-year history of diabetes
C. One with retinopathy and nephropathy
D. One with peripheral vascular disease and peripheral neuropathy

9 The most reliable indicator of thyroid dysfunction is:

A. An abnormal serum triiodothyronine level
B. An abnormal serum thyroxine (T₄) level
C. An abnormal basal metabolic rate
D. Abnormal deep tendon reflexes

10 Which assessment finding is *not* a characteristic clinical manifestation of Graves' disease?

A. Tachycardia
B. A bruit over the thyroid
C. Exophthalmos
D. Dry skin

11 Which assessment finding indicates a euthyroid state in a patient taking 100 mg of propylthiouracil (PTU) P.O. three times daily?

A. Irritability
B. Bradycardia
C. Pulse rate of 74 beats/minute
D. Increased T_4 level

12 Which measure should the nurse take before administering a patient's inital dose of propylthiouracil?

A. Checking the prothrombin time
B. Assessing vital signs
C. Performing a lupus erythematosus cell preparation
D. Performing a white blood cell count

13 Which type of diet should a patient with hypothyroidism avoid?

A. Low-sodium
B. High-cholesterol
C. Low-calorie
D. High-fiber

14 Acromegaly is primarily caused by:

A. Oversecretion of growth hormone by the posterior lobe of the pituitary
B. Oversecretion of growth hormone by the anterior lobe of the pituitary
C. Congenital deficiency in the secretion of growth hormone
D. Deficiency in the secretion of hormones by the anterior and posterior lobes of the pituitary

15 Mr. P., a patient with acromegaly, refuses to have his pituitary gland removed surgically; radiation therapy is then discussed. If the patient voices concerns about possible decreased libido, which response should the nurse make?

A. "Hormone replacement therapy will correct this problem"
B. "Since the pituitary is not involved with sex hormones, this treatment will not affect your sex drive"
C. "This treatment increases the secretion of gonadotropins, which will increase your sex drive"
D. "The posterior lobe of the pituitary is still intact, so your sex drive will not be affected"

16 The characteristic bronzed appearance of the distal extremities of a patient with Addison's disease is caused by:

A. Increased production of melanocyte-stimulating hormone (MSH)
B. Decreased production of MSH
C. Stimulation of the pituitary from a decreased blood cortisol level
D. Androgen deficiency associated with Addison's disease

17 Parenteral injections of cortisol for a patient with Addison's disease should be injected:

A. Deep into the deltoid muscle
B. Into the subcutaneous tissue
C. Deep into the gluteal muscle
D. After the patient eats

18 Before a patient with Addison's disease is discharged, the nurse should tell him that:

A. He will require short-term medical follow-up after discharge
B. He should carry an identification bracelet and an emergency kit containing hydrocortisone (Solu-Cortef)
C. He should decrease his dose of glucocorticoids when undergoing stressful conditions
D. He may need to decrease his dose of mineralocorticoids during periods of strenuous physical exertion or fever

19 A possibly malignant lump in a patient's breast can be diagnosed definitively only with:

A. Mammography
B. Needle aspiration
C. Thermography
D. Biopsy

20 According to current American Cancer Society recommendations, women age 50 and over should have a routine mammography:

A. Every year
B. Every 2 years
C. Every 5 years
D. Only if symptomatic

21

When the physician suspects breast cancer, he commonly recommends a two-stage procedure in which a biopsy is performed and treatment begins several days later. Which of the following is *not* considered an advantage of this two-stage procedure?

A. Allows patient to obtain a second opinion
B. Permits patient to participate in planning of subsequent care
C. Gives patient time to psychologically adjust to impending treatment
D. Increases long-term survival

22

Which assessment finding in a patient with prostatic cancer indicates metastasis?

A. A complaint of lumbosacral pain
B. Pus in the urine
C. Urinary frequency and decreased urinary stream
D. Decreased serum alkaline phosphatase level

23

During estrogen therapy for prostatic cancer, a patient complains of decreased libido. What is the nurse's most appropriate response?

A. "I'll report this to your physician immediately"
B. "This will disappear in a week or so"
C. "Maybe you're allergic to the drugs"
D. "This is an adverse effect of estrogen therapy"

24

Which type of penile prosthesis causes a permanent semierection?

A. Silicone rod type
B. Inflatable type
C. Hinged type
D. All of the above

25

A patient returns from surgery for the insertion of an inflatable penile prosthesis with an indwelling urinary (Foley) catheter in place. Which assessment finding should the nurse report immediately to the physician?

A. Scrotal edema and discoloration
B. Discomfort when the patient first voids
C. A bruised, swollen penis
D. Edema in the area of the fluid reservoir

26 Which assessment finding should the nurse expect in a patient with suspected pelvic inflammatory disease (PID)?

A. Upper abdominal pain
B. Spotting
C. Foul-smelling vaginal discharge
D. Hematuria

27 Which test is most reliable in diagnosing syphilis in all stages?

A. Dark-field examination
B. Venereal Disease Research Laboratory test
C. Fluorescent treponemol antibody absorption test
D. Tzanck test

28 The physician orders probenecid (Benemid) before administration of penicillin G benzathine (Bicillin L-A) I.M. to a patient with primary syphilis. Probenecid is given first to:

A. Reduce the pain associated with penicillin administration
B. Increase uric acid excretion
C. Help maintain high blood levels of penicillin
D. Delay allergic responses to penicillin

29 Which assessment finding is *not* likely in a female patient with gonorrhea?

A. Painful urination
B. Yellowish green vaginal discharge
C. Lower abdominal pain and distention
D. Rectal inflammation and discomfort

30 Which statement about herpes genitalis is *not* correct?

A. There appears to be an association between herpes and cervical cancer
B. Once treated, active immunity develops
C. The disease is spread by the oral-genital route
D. It causes painful ulcerations on the genitals

31 Acyclovir sodium (Zovirax) is used to treat herpes genitalis. Which adverse effects should the nurse assess for when administering this drug intravenously?

A. Hypertension and edema
B. Dizziness and headache
C. Arrhythmias and hypotension
D. Hematuria and polyuria

32 Which topic of discussion is *not* appropriate for a patient with a chlamydial infection?

A. Sexual partners should be treated simultaneously
B. The patient should follow the prescribed therapy for the specified time
C. Sexual activity can be resumed once treatment has been completed
D. Reevaluation cultures are needed when therapy is completed

33 The drug of choice for treating a nonpregnant woman with a chlamydial infection is:

A. Tetracycline (Achromycin)
B. Erythromycin (Erythrocin)
C. Penicillin G potassium (Pfizerpen)
D. Clindamycin (Cleocin)

SITUATION

Mr. B., age 40, has been experiencing sporadic episodes of pounding headaches, intermittent elevated blood pressures, and emotional instability. Blood tests reveal a glucose level of 350 mg/dl.

Questions 34 and 35 refer to this situation.

34 The physician orders a 24-hour urine collection for Mr. B. to check the vanillylmandelic acid (VMA) level. Before the test, the nurse should advise Mr. B. to:

A. Omit red meats from his diet for several days
B. Avoid tea, fruits, and chocolate for 3 days
C. Decrease his intake of fats and carbohydrates
D. Leave collected urine at room temperature

35 After reviewing the VMA test report, the physician diagnoses pheochromocytoma. Therefore, Mr. B.'s clinical manifestations are caused primarily by:

A. The effects of excessive catecholamines
B. The effect of the tumor mass
C. Overactivity of the parasympathetic nervous system
D. Overactivity of the adrenal cortex

SITUATION

Ms. E., a 25-year-old patient on lithium carbonate (Lithonate) therapy, begins to experience polyuria and polydipsia. She also complains of fatigue and constipation. Physical assessment reveals a blood pressure of 108/66 mm Hg and poor skin turgor. The physician diagnoses diabetes insipidus.

Questions 36 and 37 refer to this situation.

36 Which nursing intervention is *not* appropriate for Ms. E.?

A. Weighing her daily
B. Assessing the urine specific gravity every 6 hours
C. Forcing fluids
D. Assessing the urine for sugar and acetone

37 The physician orders chlorpropamide (Diabinese) for Ms. E. to:

A. Stimulate insulin secretion in the pancreas
B. Potentiate the action of antidiuretic hormone
C. Promote diuresis by decreasing the reabsorption of sodium
D. Provide active transport of insulin into the cells

SITUATION

Ms. H., age 20, is admitted to the hospital with hyperglycemia, anxiety, hypokalemia, and muscle wasting. The physician diagnoses Cushing's syndrome and orders 2 g of mitotane (Lysodren) four times daily.

Questions 38 to 41 refer to this situation.

38 The following morning, the nurse notices that Ms. H. seems depressed. This depression is probably caused by:

A. Glucocorticoid excess
B. Androgen deficiency
C. The patient's fear of a prolonged hospitalization
D. An overdose of mitotane

39 When caring for Ms. H., the nurse should:

A. Weigh her once a week
B. Keep her bed's side rails down at all times to help decrease her anxiety
C. Force fluids
D. Protect her from infection

40 The physician orders a low-calorie, low-carbohydrate, low-sodium, and high-potassium diet for Ms. H. Which statement would indicate that she understands the diet and its importance in her treatment plan?

A. "I'd like peanuts for a snack after dinner"
B. "I think I will eat fish and vegetables tonight"
C. "I won't need dinner tonight—my friend is bringing me a hamburger and french fries"
D. "My diet is important, but everyone cheats once in a while when dieting"

41 After several days of hospitalization, Ms. H.'s upper arm develops large areas of ecchymoses. This is probably from:

A. Blood pressure measurements
B. Fat redistribution
C. Steroid administration
D. Virilization

SITUATION

M., a 20-year-old student who has had insulin-dependent diabetes mellitus (IDDM) for 1 year, is admitted to the hospital for evaluation of his diabetes. He states that his blood glucose tests at home are always in the 240 to 300 mg/dl range. He takes 20 units of NPH insulin each morning and follows a 2,800-calorie diet. He is 6 feet 2 inches tall, weighs 180 lb., and has no complaints other than hyperglycemia.

Questions 42 to 47 refer to this situation.

42 Which measure should the nurse always include when developing a care plan for a patient with IDDM?

A. Deep breathing and coughing every hour
B. Assessment of consciousness level every 2 hours
C. Blood pressure measurement every 4 hours
D. Assessment of blood glucose level by fingerstick before meals and before bed

43 The physician adds regular insulin to M.'s usual morning NPH insulin dose to provide early insulin activity. Which step followed by the nurse in preparing and administering the insulin has the greatest effect on insulin activity?

A. Injecting a volume of air equal to the NPH dose into the NPH bottle
B. Drawing regular insulin into the syringe before NPH
C. Injecting the insulin immediately after mixing
D. Injecting the insulin into the abdomen

44 While planning his evening meal, M. asks the nurse why he cannot find corn on the vegetable list of his exchange diet booklet. The best response by the nurse would be:

A. "Yellow vegetables are not listed with the green vegetables"
B. "Corn is very starchy; diabetics should avoid it"
C. "Corn is a starchy vegetable; it is found in the bread and starch exchange list"
D. "Corn is a high-fiber vegetable and should be included in the diabetic diet"

45 Because M. requires insulin, he may complain of frequent headaches, irritability, hunger, excessive food intake, and weight gain resulting from:

A. Excessive insulin
B. Insufficient insulin
C. Insufficient exercise
D. Noncompliance with the prescribed diet

46 While assessing M.'s self-administration technique, the nurse observes that he injects the insulin into an area of hypertrophied tissue on the anterior thigh. Which action should the nurse take?

A. Advise the patient to switch to an insulin preparation of greater purity
B. Advise the patient to rotate insulin injection sites and avoid the hypertrophied area
C. Advise the patient to administer all insulin injections at a 90-degree angle
D. Advise the patient to consult a dermatologist about the hypertrophied tissue

47 M. tells the nurse that he plans to start a regular exercise program. What should the nurse tell him?

A. "Always eat extra food before exercising"
B. "Always reduce your insulin dosage on the days you exercise"
C. "Check your blood glucose level before and after exercising"
D. "Never engage in strenuous exercise"

SITUATION

Mr. D., an 80-year-old man with diet-controlled diabetes and a history of congestive heart failure, is admitted to the emergency department because of lethargy and twitching of his left hand and left leg. He is severely dehydrated; laboratory test results reveal a blood glucose level of 1,300 mg/dl. His wife states that he has had an upper respiratory infection and has complained of increased urination, excessive thirst, and fatigue during the past week.

Questions 48 and 49 refer to this situation.

48 The most likely diagnosis is:

A. Right-sided cerebrovascular accident
B. Absence seizures
C. Diabetic ketoacidosis
D. Hyperosmolar nonketotic syndrome

49 Because of Mr. D.'s cardiac history, the nurse should discuss which order with the physician before implementation?

A. Administration of 5 units of regular insulin I.V. immediately
B. Instillation of normal saline solution at 1,000 ml/hour
C. Blood glucose level measurements by fingerstick method every 30 minutes
D. Insertion of a central venous pressure line

SITUATION

Mr. J. and his wife have been married for 12 years and have six children. They are satisfied with the size of their family and are considering birth control measures. Mr. J. wishes to learn about vasectomy.

Questions 50 to 52 refer to this situation.

50 Because psychological preparation for a patient considering a vasectomy is important, the nurse should give Mr. J. all of the following information *except:*

A. His body will continue to produce sex hormones
B. His volume of semen will decline appreciably
C. His sexual drive should not diminish
D. He will be able to achieve and maintain an erection

51 Mr. J. undergoes a vasectomy. Which nursing measure is *not* recommended for relieving his local scrotal discomfort and swelling during the first 24 hours after the procedure?

A. Applying heat to the scrotum
B. Applying ice bags to the scrotum
C. Elevating the legs
D. Supporting the scrotum

52 Which postsurgical instruction is *not* appropriate for Mr. J.?

A. "Bring in a semen specimen every month"
B. "Avoid strenuous exercises for 5 to 7 days"
C. "You may resume intercourse in 1 week without the usual contraceptive method"
D. "You should not go to work for 2 or 3 days"

SITUATION

Mrs. R., age 48, is admitted to the hospital with complaints of menorrhagia with each menstrual cycle and heaviness in the lower abdomen. A pelvic examination reveals an enlarged uterus; a Pap smear reveals suspicious cells. The physician diagnoses uterine leiomyoma.

Questions 53 to 56 refer to this situation.

53 Which clinical manifestation besides heavy, prolonged bleeding might the nurse observe in Mrs. R.?

A. Varicosities of the lower extremities
B. Frequent episodes of diarrhea
C. Urine retention
D. Amenorrhagia

54 Because of Mrs. R.'s chronic fatigue and the progressive enlargement of the tumor, the physician schedules a total abdominal hysterectomy and bilateral salpingo-oophorectomy (TAH-BSO). Which assessment finding factor is most influential in the decision to perform a hysterectomy rather than a myomectomy on Mrs. R.?

A. The degree of bleeding
B. Size of enlargement
C. Suspicious cells on the Pap smear
D. Complaint of dyspareunia

55 Three days after the procedure, Mrs. R. complains of severe gas pain. Which drug would be most effective in relieving this gas pain?

A. Meperidine (Demerol)
B. Ranitidine (Zantac)
C. Bethanechol (Urecholine)
D. Simethicone (Mylicon)

56 Before Mrs. R.'s discharge, the nurse should caution her against:

A. Taking showers
B. Lifting heavy amounts
C. Maintaining good hydration
D. Wearing a soft girdle

SITUATION

Mrs. M., age 36, is admitted to the hospital with a tentative diagnosis of cervical cancer.

Questions 57 to 59 refer to this situation.

57 Which diagnostic test would be most conclusive in confirming invasive cervical cancer?

A. Pap smear
B. Colposcopy
C. Biopsy
D. Schiller's iodine test

58 Diagnostic testing confirms stage II b cervical cancer. The physician recommends internal radium implants and orders the insertion of an indwelling urinary (Foley) catheter before radium implantation to:

A. Prevent pressure on the sutures
B. Minimize the pain associated with the implants
C. Prevent urinary tract infection
D. Prevent bladder distention

59 After the procedure, the physician places Mrs. M. on complete bed rest. Which nursing measure is contraindicated for Mrs. M.?

A. Keeping all visitors a specific distance from the patient
B. Turning the patient periodically
C. Allowing no visitors
D. Using a room deodorizer

Answer sheet

	A B C D		A B C D
1	○ ○ ○ ○	31	○ ○ ○ ○
2	○ ○ ○ ○	32	○ ○ ○ ○
3	○ ○ ○ ○	33	○ ○ ○ ○
4	○ ○ ○ ○	34	○ ○ ○ ○
5	○ ○ ○ ○	35	○ ○ ○ ○
6	○ ○ ○ ○	36	○ ○ ○ ○
7	○ ○ ○ ○	37	○ ○ ○ ○
8	○ ○ ○ ○	38	○ ○ ○ ○
9	○ ○ ○ ○	39	○ ○ ○ ○
10	○ ○ ○ ○	40	○ ○ ○ ○
11	○ ○ ○ ○	41	○ ○ ○ ○
12	○ ○ ○ ○	42	○ ○ ○ ○
13	○ ○ ○ ○	43	○ ○ ○ ○
14	○ ○ ○ ○	44	○ ○ ○ ○
15	○ ○ ○ ○	45	○ ○ ○ ○
16	○ ○ ○ ○	46	○ ○ ○ ○
17	○ ○ ○ ○	47	○ ○ ○ ○
18	○ ○ ○ ○	48	○ ○ ○ ○
19	○ ○ ○ ○	49	○ ○ ○ ○
20	○ ○ ○ ○	50	○ ○ ○ ○
21	○ ○ ○ ○	51	○ ○ ○ ○
22	○ ○ ○ ○	52	○ ○ ○ ○
23	○ ○ ○ ○	53	○ ○ ○ ○
24	○ ○ ○ ○	54	○ ○ ○ ○
25	○ ○ ○ ○	55	○ ○ ○ ○
26	○ ○ ○ ○	56	○ ○ ○ ○
27	○ ○ ○ ○	57	○ ○ ○ ○
28	○ ○ ○ ○	58	○ ○ ○ ○
29	○ ○ ○ ○	59	○ ○ ○ ○
30	○ ○ ○ ○		

Answers and rationales

1 Correct answer—**B**

Kussmaul's respirations are deep, rapid breaths characteristic of diabetic ketoacidosis (DKA); they indicate that the body is trying to compensate for the acidotic state by eliminating greater amounts of carbon dioxide. DKA, an acute complication of diabetes in adults, results from insufficient insulin relative to glucose and excess counterregulatory hormones; hyperglycemia and incomplete fat metabolism follows, causing excessive ketones. Clinical manifestations include polyuria and polydipsia leading to profound dehydration, fatigue, lethargy, and possibly coma. Hyperosmolar nonketotic syndrome (HNKS) is another complication of diabetes mellitus that elevates the serum glucose level but does not cause excessive ketone production; respirations with HNKS are characteristically shallow and rapid. Gastroparesis, or delayed stomach emptying, is a sign of diabetic autonomic neuropathy, a chronic complication of diabetes; common clinical manifestations include nausea, vomiting, bloating, and anorexia. Glomerulosclerosis refers to progressive deterioration of the glomeruli of the kidney; this chronic complication of diabetes leads to renal failure.

2 Correct answer—**C**

Diazoxide (Hyperstat) is a benzothiadiazide that causes hyperglycemia by inhibiting insulin secretion; it is used to treat hypoglycemia caused by excessive insulin production. Chlorpropamide (Diabinese), glipizide (Glucotrol), and tolbutamide (Orinase) are oral hypoglycemic agents used to treat Type II (non-insulin-dependent) diabetes mellitus. Chlorpropamide and tolbutamide are first-generation sulfonylureas that have been used extensively since 1965. Glipizide is a second-generation sulfonylurea approved for use in the United States in 1984; this medication is more potent than the first-generation ones and is associated with fewer complications.

3 Correct answer—**B**

Diabetes control worsens with the use of prednisone (Deltasone), a glucocorticoid and insulin antagonist. This drug increases glucose production by the liver and inhibits glucose use by the peripheral tissues; therefore, it increases the blood glucose level in a diabetic patient and impairs diabetes control. Prednisone therapy may cause frequent hyperglycemic, not hypoglycemic, reactions by increasing blood glucose levels.

4 Correct answer—**D**

Weight reduction in a newly diagnosed obese adult with Type II diabetes improves blood glucose levels and often eliminates the need for antidiabetic agents. This effect of weight loss on blood glucose levels may result from increased insulin secretion by the pancreas, enhanced insulin action at peripheral tissues, and decreased glucose production by the liver. Blood glucose monitoring shows the effects of food, exercise, and stress on blood glucose levels, but it does not improve those levels. Avoiding sugar-containing foods completely and adhering strictly to the American Diabetes Association exchange diet are not always necessary if the patient can lose weight and lower blood glucose levels without these measures.

5 Correct answer—**B**

Daily early-morning elevations in blood glucose after normal daytime blood glucose levels are a common response to a single morning injection of an intermediate insulin, such as isophane insulin suspension (NPH), resulting from insulin depletion during the night; it can be corrected by administering additional NPH before dinner or at bedtime. Excessive evening snacks are not the most likely cause of morning hyperglycemia because blood glucose elevations caused by food eaten the previous night usually resolve by morning. The dawn phenomenon is an early-morning elevation in blood glucose resulting from the secretion of growth hormone. This insulin antagonist is secreted during sleep, and its anti-insulin effect is experienced 6 hours later; however, because this hormonal secretion varies from day to day, dawn phenomenon does not occur on a daily basis. Rebound hyperglycemia refers to elevated morning blood glucose levels after insulin-induced nighttime hypoglycemia; it usually results from an excessive morning insulin dose. Because rebound hyperglycemia also causes elevations in blood glucose levels despite increased insulin dosage and subtle clinical signs of nighttime hypoglycemia (such as evening and morning headaches), it would not be the cause of the patient's early-morning hyperglycemia.

6 Correct answer—**D**

Health care professionals commonly assume that poor diabetes control results from deliberate noncompliance with the prescribed treatment, but many patients have never received diabetes education or were taught but did not learn the essential aspects of diabetes care; therefore, problems with diabetes control may result from the patient's inadequate knowledge and incorrect management skills rather than noncompliance. Assessment identifies the need for education and the areas in which education should focus. Exploring the reason for noncompliance, arranging a family conference, and teaching about complications should be considered only after lack of knowledge and management skills are ruled out as the cause of poor diabetes control.

7 Correct answer—C

This elevation in blood glucose probably results from rebound hyperglycemia. A hypoglycemic episode from any cause is usually followed by a release of counterregulatory hormones, including glucagon, cortisol, growth hormone, and catecholamines; as a result, glucose production by the liver increases, glucose utilization by muscle tissue is inhibited, and blood glucose levels rise. At times, this hormonal response to glucose is prolonged and exaggerated; it is then called rebound hyperglycemia, or the Somogyi phenomenon. Excessive orange juice is not the most likely cause of morning hyperglycemia; 6 oz of orange juice contain 15 g of glucose, the standard recommended treatment for hypoglycemia. Insufficient insulin commonly causes early-morning hyperglycemia in patients receiving one dose of an intermediate insulin, but the hypoglycemic reaction at 2 a.m. rules this out as the cause of hyperglycemia in this situation. Because the dawn phenomenon, an early-morning rise in blood glucose caused by the secretion of growth hormone, is not usually preceded by hypoglycemia, it is also an unlikely cause in this case.

8 Correct answer—D

All diabetic patients should follow a daily foot care regimen, but it is particularly important for one with peripheral vascular disease and peripheral neuropathy because of the increased risk of serious foot disease. The absence of sensation associated with peripheral neuropathy may prevent the patient from noticing the development of injuries, calluses, or pressure points of the toes and metatarsal heads; ischemia caused by progressively diminishing circulation to the lower extremities prevents healing and greatly increases the patient's risk of developing infection and gangrene.

9 Correct answer—B

The most reliable indicator of thyroid dysfunction is an abnormal thyroxine (T_4) level. T_4 is a hormone produced and stored in the thyroid gland until released into the bloodstream in response to thyroid-stimulating hormone; in almost all patients with thyroid dysfunction, the serum T_4 level is abnormal. Triidothyronine (T_3) is also a thyroid hormone, but it is much less stable than T_4 and is produced in much smaller amounts; therefore, the serum T_3 level is a less reliable indicator of thyroid dysfunction than the T_4 level. Although thyroid hormones influence the rate of oxygen consumption, the basal metabolic rate (BMR) does not indicate thyroid dysfunction as accurately as the serum T_4 level; BMR changes may be caused by other disorders, such as infection and malnutrition. Abnormal deep tendon reflexes may result from thyroid dysfunction or from hypothermia, peripheral neuropathy, and other disorders unrelated to thyroid function; therefore, they are not a reliable indicator of thyroid disorder.

10 Correct answer—D

Dry skin is not a characteristic clinical manifestation of Graves' disease. Excessive T_4 and T_3 secretion increases the BMR, resulting in increased cardiac activity, or tachycardia. This in turn increases blood flow, causing a bruit over the thyroid. The increased BMR also raises heat production, leading to heat intolerance. Exophthalmos—abnormal protrusion of the eyes—develops in 75% of patients with Graves' disease but is rare in hyperthyroidism with other causes; it may result from the accumulation of fluid in the fat pads and muscles behind the eyeballs.

11 Correct answer—C

A pulse rate of 74 beats/minute is within the normal range, indicating normal activity of the thyroid gland (euthyroid state). Irritability would indicate a hyperthyroid state. Bradycardia—a pulse rate less than 60 beats/minute—would indicate a hypothyroid state. A decreased T_4 level, not an increased one, would indicate an euthyroid state.

12 Correct answer—D

Propylthiouracil (PTU) commonly causes agranulocytosis; by taking a baseline white blood cell (WBC) count and periodic WBC counts after drug therapy begins, the nurse can detect developing agranulocytosis, which predisposes the patient to fulminating infection. Checking the patient's prothrombin time would provide no useful information because PTU does not affect clotting. Taking vital signs, particularly the temperature, would be more appropriate after drug therapy has started, to detect infection at an early stage. The lupus erythematosus (LE) cell preparation is used to diagnose LE, a collagen disease.

13 Correct answer—B

Hypothyroidism causes abnormalities in cholesterol and triglyceride metabolism, predisposing the patient to atherosclerosis and arteriosclerosis; cholesterol intake should be low to prevent these conditions. A low-sodium diet is recommended because sodium may contribute to cardiac disease. The patient's diet should be low in calories because hypothyroidism lowers the metabolic rate. A high fiber intake also is recommended because most high-fiber foods are low in calories; high-fiber foods also stimulate peristalsis, which prevents constipation.

14 Correct answer—B

Acromegaly, a condition that occurs in adults, is caused primarily by oversecretion of growth hormone produced by the anterior lobe of the pituitary. (In children, this condition is called gigantism.) The posterior lobe of the pituitary secretes antidiuretic hormone (ADH) and oxytoxin, not growth hormone. A congenital deficiency in the secretion of growth hormone results in dwarfism. Insufficient hormone secretion by the posterior and anterior lobes causes panhypopituitarism; this condition has many more clinical manifestations than acromegaly, including GI disturbances, symptoms of Addison's disease with less skin pigmentation, deficient thyroid function, and decreased BMR.

15 Correct answer—A

The nurse should reassure the patient that hormone replacement therapy will correct any decrease in libido caused by radiation therapy. The anterior lobe of the pituitary is involved with sex hormone production; radiation therapy affects the sex drive by causing decreased, not increased, hormone secretion. The posterior lobe of the gland produces ADH and oxytoxin, which are not related to the sex drive.

16 Correct answer—A

Addison's disease causes increased, not decreased, secretion of melanocyte-stimulating hormone (MSH), which results in increased pigmentation of the skin and mucous membranes; this hyperpigmentation is reversed with treatment. Addison's disease causes decreased, not increased, blood cortisol level; this decreased level stimulates the pituitary, which increases MSH secretion. The androgen deficiency associated with the disease causes decreased libido and loss of axillary and pubic hair; this effect is marked in men because testicular androgens exert the major androgenic metabolic effects.

17 Correct answer—C

Because sufficient muscle mass is necessary for accurate injection of parenteral cortisol preparations, the nurse should inject them deep into the gluteal muscle, not into the smaller deltoid muscle.

Cortisol should not be injected subcutaneously because this may cause sterile abscesses, tissue atrophy, and pigmentation abnormalities. Steroid therapy causes GI disturbances with oral administration, not I.M. injection; therefore, the patient does not need to have food in his stomach before administration.

18 Correct answer—B

The patient with Addison's disease should wear an identification bracelet that lists his adrenal insufficiency along with the name and phone number of his physician; he should also carry an emergency kit containing hydrocortisone (Solu-Cortef) for injection if trauma, vomiting, loss of consciousness, or another serious condition occurs. This disease requires daily medication and life-long medical follow-up to control it. Stressful conditions require higher levels of glucocorticoids to maintain normal glycemic states; the patient should call his physician during these times for instructions on increasing doses. Mineralocorticoids may need to be increased temporarily to maintain fluid and electrolyte balance during periods of profuse diaphoresis, such as strenuous physical exertion and fever.

19 Correct answer—D

The only diagnostic test considered 100% accurate is biopsy, which may be incisional (part of the lesion is surgically removed) or excisional (the entire lesion is surgically removed). Mammography is valuable as a screening measure, but it does not differentiate between benign and malignant lesions. Needle aspiration helps diagnose a fluid-filled cyst, but it does not diagnose a solid neoplasm; also, many physicians prefer to remove the entire lesion because needle aspiration may cause the release of malignant cells into the circulation and lymphatic system. Thermography, which uses infrared photography to detect lesions, cannot differentiate between benign and malignant lumps; according to the American College of Radiology, health care personnel should not even use this procedure as a screening test for breast cancer because it cannot detect small or deep lesions.

20 Correct answer—A

Because the risk of breast cancer begins to rise at age 40 and progressively increases through age 80, all women age 50 and over should follow the American Cancer Society recommendation for yearly mammography examinations.

21 Correct answer—D

Evidence indicates that a delay of up to 4 days between biopsy and treatment neither increases nor decreases the long-term survival rate. If the biopsy reveals a malignant neoplasm, the patient has time to obtain a second opinion, participate in planning subsequent care, and psychologically adjust to the impending treatment.

22 Correct answer—A

A complaint of lumbosacral pain indicates metastasis; the most common form of metastasis by the hematogenous route is osseous, and the most common sites are the pelvis, lumbar spine, and ribs. Pus in the urine indicates urinary tract infection, not metastasis. Urinary frequency and decreased urinary stream are caused by urinary obstruction, not metastasis. The serum alkaline phosphatase level would be elevated, not decreased, with metastasis as a result of increased bone activity.

23 Correct answer—D

The nurse should provide information explaining the cause of decreased libido; therefore, stating that it is an adverse effect of estrogen therapy in male patients is the most appropriate response. Because this adverse effect is common, the nurse does not need to alert the physician immediately. The nurse should not tell the patient that this effect will resolve itself shortly; it will persist as long as estrogen therapy continues. Decreased libido is not an allergic response.

24 Correct answer—A

The silicone rod is the least expensive penile prosthesis and the simplest to implant; its major disadvantage is that it is semirigid, causing the penis to remain partially erect at all times. An inflatable penile prosthesis simulates natural flaccidity and erection by means of a small bulb pump in the scrotum and a reservoir of fluid in the abdomen. Hinged prostheses are used in the extremities, not the penis.

25 Correct answer—D

Edema in the area of the fluid reservoir indicates spillage of the radiopaque fluid into the abdomen; the nurse should report this finding to the physician immediately. Scrotal edema and discoloration, discomfort when the patient first voids, and a bruised, swollen penis are expected findings after this procedure.

26 Correct answer—C

The nurse should expect a foul-smelling vaginal discharge in a patient with suspected pelvic inflammatory disease (PID); the discharge may be purulent if caused by gonorrhea. PID causes pain in the lower abdomen, not the upper abdomen. Spotting and hematuria are not associated with PID.

27 Correct answer—C

The most reliable test in diagnosing syphilis in all stages is the fluorescent treponemol antibody absorption test, which identifies antigens of the causative spirochete *Treponema pallidum* in tissue, exudates, and secretions. A dark-field examination can identify the spirochete effectively only when moist lesions are present, as in primary, secondary, and prenatal syphilis. The Venereal Disease Research Laboratory test is not conclusive because it commonly gives false-positive results, particularly in patients with collagen diseases, hepatitis, and infectious mononucleosis. The Tzanck test is used to diagnose herpes genitalis, not syphilis.

28 Correct answer—C

Probenecid (Benemid) delays renal excretion of penicillin; it is given before penicillin G benzathine (Bicillin L-A) to help maintain high blood levels of penicillin, which are necessary when treating syphilis. Probenecid is not an analgesic; it does not decrease the pain associated with I.M. injection. The drug increases uric acid excretion, but that is not the reason for its use in this situation; syphilis is not related to uric acid levels. Patients allergic to penicillin are given tetracycline instead.

29 Correct answer—B

Vaginal discharge is not common in the female patient with gonorrhea, although the male patient with gonorrhea typically has a yellowish green, cloudy penile discharge. Painful urination may occur if the urethra is involved. Lower abdominal pain and distention, which result from pelvic inflammation, are common. Rectal inflammation and discomfort are also typical.

30 Correct answer—B

Herpes genitalis can recur after treatment; immunity to the virus does not develop. Although not definite, a link between herpes and cervical cancer appears to exist. The disease is spread by oral-genital route and causes painful vesicles and ulceration of the genitals.

The patient may require counseling and psychological support to cope with this prognosis. Herpes genitalis should not interfere with resuming sexual contact with appropriate precautions, including the use of a condom if the partner does not have the disease and abstinence when lesions are present. Stress, sunburn, and tight clothing can trigger a recurrence by creating extra warmth in the genital area.

31 Correct answer—B

The nurse should assess for dizziness and headache when administering acyclovir sodium (Zovirax) intravenously. Because the drug causes renal damage, the patient may develop hematuria, edema, and oliguria (not polyuria). Hypotension may occur, but the drug does not cause arrhythmias or hypertension.

32 Correct answer—D

The Centers for Disease Control recommends 1 week of antibiotic treatment for the patient with chlamydia but does not recommend reevaluation cultures after therapy. All sexual partners should be treated simultaneously to prevent reinfection. Because the infection is sexually transmitted by *Chlamydia trachomatis,* an organism that can remain in the genital tract asymptomatically, the patient should follow the prescribed therapy for the specified time even if symptoms disappear earlier. Once treatment has been completed, the patient may resume sexual activity.

33 Correct answer—A

The drug of choice for treating a nonpregnant woman with a chlamydial infection is tetracycline (Achromycin); however, erythromycin (Erythrocin) is the drug of choice for a pregnant woman because it does not have tetracycline's teratogenic effect on the fetus. Because penicillin G potassium (Pfizerpen) is effective against only gram-positive bacillus, it has no effect on *Chlamydia trachomatis,* a gram-negative bacteria. Clindamycin (Cleocin) is not effective against chlamydial infections; it is used only to treat infections caused by staphylococci and streptococci.

34 Correct answer—B

Tea, fruits, and chocolate are high in catecholamines; because vanillylmandelic acid (VMA) is a catecholamine metabolite, the patient should avoid these foods for 3 days before the test to prevent inaccuracies. Avoiding red meats is necessary before obtaining a fecal specimen for occult blood, not a urine specimen for VMA testing. Fat and carbohydrate intake does not affect VMA levels. Collected urine should be refrigerated or kept on ice to prevent inaccuracies in the test.

35 Correct answer—A

A pheochromocytoma is a tumor of the adrenal medulla that secretes the catecholamines epinephrine and norepinephrine; the patient's clinical manifestations primarily result from excessive amounts of catecholamines, which cause vasoconstriction. These manifestations do not result from effects of the tumor mass. Overactivity of the parasympathetic nervous system would cause increased acetylcholine release, resulting in vasodilation instead of vasoconstriction. The adrenal cortex secretes glucose, mineralocorticoids, and androgens; overactivity would not change catecholamine levels or cause vasoconstriction.

36 Correct answer—D

Assessing the patient's urine for sugar and acetone is inappropriate because her condition is not related to incomplete metabolism of fats or carbohydrates. Because diabetes insipidus causes a deficiency in antidiuretic hormone (ADH), the patient's urine output is chronically increased; therefore, the nurse should force fluids to replace those lost, weigh the patient daily to assess fluid loss, and assess the urine specific gravity frequently to determine urine concentration.

37 Correct answer—B

The physician orders chlorpropamide (Diabinese) for this patient to potentiate the action of ADH, which helps reverse diuresis. This drug stimulates the insulin secretion from the pancreas, but this action helps treat diabetes mellitus, not diabetes insipidus. Chlorpropamide does not affect sodium reabsorption or provide active transport of insulin.

38 Correct answer—A

Cushing's syndrome causes excessive glucocorticoids, which typically results in emotional lability and other mental changes. Cushing's syndrome does not cause androgen deficiency. The patient with this disorder typically is not hospitalized for long. Mitotane (Lysodren), which decreases glucocorticoid levels, is extremely toxic to the adrenal cortex and may cause depression; however, overdose is not likely because the ordered dosage is within the recommended dosage of 2 to 16 g daily.

39 Correct answer—D

Glucocorticoid excess inhibits both humoral immunity and cell-mediated immunity, which can lead to bacterial and viral infections; the nurse should take basic precautions, such as washing hands thoroughly, to prevent infection. The nurse should weigh the patient daily to assess for edema as well as congestive heart failure resulting from sodium retention. The bed's side rails should be up at all times to prevent falls; glucocorticoid excess weakens the protein matrix of bones, increasing the risk of fractures from falling. Forced fluids, combined with the sodium retention caused by Cushing's syndrome, would increase the risk of fluid overload.

40 Correct answer—B

Vegetables and fish are high in potassium and reasonably low in calories and sodium. The patient should not eat peanuts, which are high in sodium. Hamburgers and french fries, which are high in calories, carbohydrates, and sodium, are prohibited. Stating everyone cheats occasionally indicates that the patient does not understand how vital proper diet is in treating Cushing's syndrome.

41 Correct answer—A

Glucocorticoid excess causes thinning of the blood vessel walls and weakening of perivascular supporting tissue, which can lead to easy bruising; therefore, the blood pressure cuff used during assessment probably caused these bruises. Fat redistribution causes truncal obesity, thinning of the extremities, and purplish striae, but not easy bruising. The patient with Cushing's syndrome is not given steroids. Virilization, or masculinization, causes such changes as hirsutism, enlarged clitoris, and atrophied breasts, but not easy bruising.

42 Correct answer—D

The nurse should assess the patient's blood glucose level by fingerstick before meals and before bed to monitor blood glucose levels and the effects of insulin administration. Deep breathing and coughing and assessing level of consciousness and blood pressure may be included in any patient's care plan, depending on the patient's particular nursing needs; however, they are not always necessary for the patient with insulin-dependent diabetes mellitus (IDDM).

43 Correct answer—C

NPH insulin contains the protein protamine, which delays the absorption of insulin; when NPH and regular insulin remain mixed in the same syringe for longer than 5 minutes, regular insulin binds to the excess protamine in the NPH and becomes slower acting, thereby losing its early activity. Injecting a volume of air equal to the NPH dose and drawing up regular insulin before the NPH are correct steps when mixing insulin in the same syringe; however, they affect the accuracy of the dose, not the activity of insulin. Injecting insulin into sites on the abdomen enhances insulin absorption and may result in earlier insulin activity, but this effect is not as significant as that achieved by injecting the insulin immediately after mixing it.

44 Correct answer—C

Because corn is a starchy vegetable, it is found on the bread and starch exchange list. One-third of a cup of corn has 68 calories and 15 g of carbohydrates, the equivalent of one slice of bread; in contrast, one-half cup of a vegetable from the vegetable exchange list contains only 28 calories and 5 g of carbohydrates. Each exchange list contains foods similar in calorie and nutritional value; they are not listed according to color or any other quality. The patient with diabetes may eat corn, but he must include it in his diet as a starchy food and determine portion size accurately. Stating that corn has a high fiber content and should be included in the diet is not incorrect, but it is not the nurse's best response in this situation because it does not answer the patient's question.

45 Correct answer—A

Insulin is an anabolic hormone that causes food to be stored as fat; excessive insulin in the circulation may cause signs of hypoglycemia, such as headaches, irritability, hunger, excessive food intake, and weight gain. The other choices would lead to elevated blood glucose levels, polyuria, and polydipsia—the cardinal signs of hyperglycemia.

46 Correct answer—B

The nurse should advise the patient to rotate insulin injection sites and to avoid the hypertrophied area. This patient has lipohypertrophy, an increased deposition of adipose tissue at the site of insulin administration, which results from insulin promoting fat storage in adipose tissue as well as trauma and scarring from repeated injections in the same area; it can lead to insulin management problems because absorption may be impaired in these areas. Lipohypertrophy does not appear to be affected by a more purified insulin preparation; however, lipoatrophy—a loss of subcutaneous fat or dimpling at injection sites—is considered an immune response to contaminants in the insulin preparation and calls for a more highly purified insulin. The angle of injection is not a factor in the development of lipohypertrophy as long as insulin is injected into the subcutaneous tissue. Rotating injection sites and avoiding the hypertrophied area usually resolve lipohypertrophy; further medical consultation should not be necessary.

47 Correct answer—C

The effects of exercise vary among patients depending on the type and intensity of exercise, the treatment method, and the patient's history of diabetes control; by testing blood glucose before and after exercise, the patient helps determine if additional food is needed or if the insulin dosage should be reduced. Telling the patient to eat additional food or reduce his insulin dosage without determining the effect of exercise on the blood glucose level may negate some of the benefits of exercise, particularly those related to weight loss and blood glucose control. Strenuous exercise is not contraindicated as long as the patient has medical clearance to exercise and the duration and intensity of exercise is increased gradually.

48 Correct answer—D

Hyperosmolar nonketotic syndrome (HNKS) is an acute complication of diabetes common in adults over age 65. It involves hyperglycemia, hyperosmolality with an extremely high blood glucose level, and intravascular volume depletion without the development of ketosis. Precipitating causes of HNKS include acute or chronic illness as well as medications that are insulin antagonists, such as propranolol (Inderal) or glucocorticoids. Symptoms of polyuria and polydipsia develop over a period of several days and neurologic findings, including coma, are typically present. Diabetic ketoacidosis is more commonly observed in younger individuals with IDDM. It develops over a brief period and is always accompanied by ketosis, which leads to metabolic acidosis. Patients with HNKS are often initially misdiagnosed as having a neurologic disorder; however, this patient's history and laboratory test results rule out cerebrovascular accident and absence seizures as the most likely diagnosis.

49 Correct answer—B

Because of the patient's cardiac history, the nurse should discuss the order for instillation of normal saline solution at 1,000 ml/hour with the physician. Normal saline solution, which is isotonic, is appropriate because the patient with HNKS should be hydrated to reverse the hyperosmolar state. However, the rate may be too fast. Many practitioners may give as much as 6 to 24 liters in the first 48 hours, but the physician may need to reduce the volume for this patient because of the potential for pulmonary edema resulting from heart dysfunction. The administration of regular insulin is necessary to reduce the high blood glucose level. The nurse should check the patient's blood glucose level frequently; glucose monitoring strips by fingerstick, which can be read visually or by a machine, are a quick, reliable way to do this. The insertion of a central venous pressure line allows accurate monitoring of fluid balance.

50 Correct answer—B

After a vasectomy, the patient's semen volume remains almost unchanged because only 0.5 ml of the total ejaculate consists of spermatozoa. The nurse should tell him that his sex hormone production, sexual interest, and ability to maintain an erection will not be affected to reassure him that the surgery will not change his masculinity.

51 Correct answer—A

The nurse should not apply heat to relieve scrotal discomfort and swelling in the first 24 hours after the patient's vasectomy; its vasodilatory effect may cause more bleeding. Ice packs, elevation of the legs, and scrotal support will help relieve the patient's discomfort.

52 Correct answer—C

The results of the vasectomy are not immediate; the patient should use another contraceptive measure until azoospermia (absence of spermatozoa in the semen) occurs. Usually, fifteen to twenty ejaculations are needed to flush remaining spermatozoa out of the vas deferens; the patient should provide a semen specimen at specified intervals to determine whether sperm are absent. Avoiding strenuous exercise for 5 to 7 days and taking 2 or 3 days off from work allows the surgical site to heal, decreasing the risk of injury and infection.

53 Correct answer—A

Varicosities of the lower extremities are a possible clinical manifestation of uterine leiomyoma, particularly if the tumor is large and located in the lower pubic region, because the tumor causes compression of muscle tissue and blood vessels. The disorder may cause constipation, not diarrhea. Urinary frequency rather than urine retention may be present because of pressure on the bladder.

Amenorrhagia is not a common clinical manifestation of uterine leiomyoma.

54 Correct answer—C

A Pap smear, although inconclusive, identifies possible precancerous or cancerous cells; if the tumor was malignant and invasive, a myomectomy might not remove all the malignant cells. A hysterectomy and bilateral salpingo-oophorectomy would be more appropriate in this case. Excessive bleeding by itself does not indicate a hysterectomy rather than a myomectomy. The size of the enlargement influences whether an abdominal or a vaginal approach is used. Dyspareunia (pain during intercourse) is not an indication for a hysterectomy.

55 Correct answer—D

The most effective drug for relieving postsurgical gas is simethicone (Mylicon); this surfactant's defoaming action breaks up mucussurrounded gas pockets in the GI tract so that they can be easily removed by belching or passing flatus. Meperidine (Demerol) is a narcotic analgesic that reduces gastric motility; doses large enough to reduce gastric secretion of hydrochloric acid might increase the difficulty of passing flatus. Bethanechol (Urecholine) increases peristaltic action of the GI tract but does not relieve gas. Ranitidine (Zantac) is a histamine$_2$-receptor inhibitor; this drug blocks the production of gastric acid secretion but does not help remove flatus.

56 Correct answer—B

The nurse should caution the patient against lifting heavy amounts after discharge because it raises intra-abdominal pressure, increasing the risk of wound disruption. Showers are not contraindicated. Good hydration is necessary to minimize hemoconcentration and decrease the risk of thrombus formation. Wearing a soft girdle provides physical and psychological support.

57 Correct answer—C

The most conclusive diagnostic test for invasive cervical cancer is a biopsy. A Pap smear typically indicates possible precancerous or cancerous epithelial cells, although it may occasionally identify cancer in situ. A colposcopy is an examination of the vagina and cervix using a magnifying lens; although helpful in locating abnormalities, it does not diagnose them conclusively. Schiller's iodine test can identify unhealthy cervical epithelium; a positive test result suggests a neoplasm but does not confirm invasive cervical cancer.

58 Correct answer—D

The indwelling urinary (Foley) catheter is inserted before internal (uterine) radium implants to prevent urine retention, which could distend the bladder and cause contact with the radioactive implants. Sutures are not needed for internal radium implants. Pain from the implants, if present, is relieved with an analgesic, not a catheter. The catheter does not prevent urinary tract infection; it increases the patient's risk of developing it.

59 Correct answer—C

Allowing the patient no visitors would not be therapeutic; because radioactive safety precautions are needed, the patient will probably feel isolated without some contact with family and friends. However, visitors must follow certain safety precautions, such as staying a specific distance from the patient and visiting for limited periods. Because the patient is on complete bed rest, she requires periodic position changes to prevent complications of bed rest by promoting circulation, enhancing lung expansion, and stimulating peristalsis. The nurse should place a deodorizer in the patient's room to minimize the odor from vaginal discharge.

CHAPTER 8

Hematologic and Immunologic Systems

Questions

1 Which type of granulocyte is produced in large numbers for phago-cytosis with a parasitic infection?

A. Monocytes
B. Eosinophils
C. Basophils
D. Neutrophils

2 Which blood cells are the first line of defense against infection of a skin laceration?

A. Neutrophils
B. Eosinophils
C. Erythrocytes
D. Platelets

3 A 29-year-old hospital worker is given immune serum globulin as prophylaxis after exposure to hepatitis B. The injection provides:

A. Natural passive immunity
B. Passive immunity
C. Natural immunity
D. Active immunity

4 All of the following are forms of active immunity *except:*

A. Rubella contact resulting in a 1:16 titer
B. Antivenoms for snake or insect bites
C. Exposure to mumps at an early age
D. Measles, mumps, and rubella vaccination

5 Which emergency treatment should the nurse perform first for a pa-tient with anaphylactic bronchospasms?

A. High Fowler's position
B. Epinephrine administration
C. Sodium bicarbonate administration
D. Oxygen therapy

6 Forty-eight hours after an intracutaneous tuberculin test, the injection site is reddened and swollen with 12-mm induration. The nurse should suspect that the:

A. Results are not clinically significant
B. Patient has allergies
C. Patient has tuberculosis
D. Patient has been exposed to *Mycobacterium tuberculosis*

7 Which blood cells produce immunoglobulins (antibodies)?

A. B lymphocytes
B. T lymphocytes
C. Macrophages
D. Neutrophils

8 Mr. H., a 40-year-old patient with Hodgkin's disease, is being treated with cyclophosphamide (Cytoxan). Which instruction would be appropriate for him?

A. "Increase your intake of raw vegetables and fruits"
B. "Brush with a firm-bristled toothbrush after each meal"
C. "Avoid people with colds or other infections"
D. "Avoid using lotions and soaps"

9 Which assessment finding is *not* a common clinical manifestation of systemic lupus erythematosus?

A. Tophi
B. Fever
C. Malaise
D. Joint problems

10 Cellulitis is a:

A. Diffuse inflammatory reaction involving cellular or connective tissue
B. Form of cellular death caused by hypoxia
C. Localized inflammatory response with a purulent exudate
D. Form of hyperplasia caused by excessive catabolism

SITUATION

Mrs. S., a 26-year-old pregnant homemaker with a 3-year-old daughter, comes to the prenatal clinic with complaints of chronic fatigue and dyspnea upon exertion. She states that she sometimes feels her heart beat rapidly. Assessment reveals extreme pallor and mild glossitis. The physician suspects iron deficiency anemia.

Questions 11 and 12 refer to this situation.

11 Which diagnostic test is most useful in confirming a diagnosis of iron deficiency anemia?

A. Erythrocyte indices
B. Total erythrocyte count
C. Hemoglobin test
D. Hematocrit test

12 The physician prescribes ferrous sulfate (Feosol) tablets for Mrs. S. to take at home twice a day. Which information should the nurse give her about this iron preparation?

A. It will turn her stools black
B. It may stain her teeth
C. It will concentrate her urine
D. It may leave a metallic aftertaste in her mouth

SITUATION

Mr. J., a 50-year-old man with a history of alcohol abuse, is brought to the hospital after being found on the street. He appears thin, weak, pale, and short of breath; he constantly shivers and complains of tingling and numbness of his fingers. Assessment reveals several ulcers on his left leg. An immediate complete blood count (CBC) reveals an abnormally high erythrocyte count (305,000,000/mm³) and mild leukopenia. The physician suspects folic acid (vitamin B₉) deficiency anemia.

Questions 13 to 16 refer to this situation.

13 To distinguish between folic acid deficiency anemia and pernicious (vitamin B_{12} deficiency) anemia, the physician orders a Schilling test to check Mr. J.'s GI absorption of vitamin B_{12}. Before the test, the nurse should instruct Mr. J. to:

A. Drink at least eight glasses of water
B. Remain in his room to protect others from radiation exposure
C. Save all but the first urine specimen for the next 24 hours
D. Save all but the first and last urine specimens for the next 24 hours

14 Which assessment finding is *not* a clinical manifestation of folic acid deficiency anemia?

A. Incoordination and weakness of the extremities
B. A sore, beefy tongue
C. Anorexia and nausea
D. Tachycardia

15 The physician orders 3 to 4 liters/minute of oxygen via nasal cannula for Mr. J. Which nursing action would *not* be appropriate during oxygen therapy?

A. Changing the cannula according to institutional policy
B. Humidifying the oxygen
C. Assessing for increased hypoxia
D. Removing the cannula during meals for greater comfort

16 Which foods are the best sources of folic acid?

A. Green, leafy vegetables and eggs
B. Kidney beans and chicken
C. Liver and asparagus
D. Carrots and fish

SITUATION

Mr. R., a 47-year-old house painter, complains of general malaise off and on for the past 6 months. He has a history of sporadic nosebleeds and of bruises after minor trauma. The nosebleeds were originally treated with cauterization and vitamin K. However, 6 months later, purpura and a few petechiae appeared on his trunk and ankles, prompting a thorough hematologic evaluation. Because of Mr. R.'s prolonged bleeding time and increased iron-binding capacity, the physician admits him to the hospital and schedules a bone marrow examination to assess for aplastic anemia.

Questions 17 to 23 refer to this situation.

17 Which intervention should the nurse implement to prevent a hematoma after bone marrow aspiration?

A. Position the patient on the aspiration site
B. Apply ice packs as ordered
C. Keep a bandage in place for 24 hours
D. Clean the site with povidone-iodine solution

18 Bone marrow aspiration reveals pancytopenia and fatty marrow, confirming aplastic anemia. Because of Mr. R.'s granulocytopenia, the nurse should try to prevent:

A. Hemorrhage
B. Bruises
C. Infection
D. Fatigue

19 Because Mr. R.'s condition probably is a result of exposure to a myelotoxic substance, blood transfusion is the preferred therapy. Mr. R. has type AB blood. Which statement about type AB blood is *not* correct?

A. The red blood cells contain A and B agglutinogens
B. The plasma is free of anti-A and anti-B agglutinins
C. Individuals with type AB blood are universal blood recipients
D. The plasma contains anti-A and anti-B agglutinins

20 Which nursing action has the highest priority when administering blood products?

A. Ensuring the correct blood product is given to the correct recipient
B. Explaining the procedure to the patient
C. Assessing for fluid overload
D. Using the appropriate filter tubing

21 The nurse should not give the patient lactated Ringer's solution before administering a unit of blood because this solution:

A. May cause hemolysis of blood
B. Has a greater osmolality than blood
C. Contains calcium, which may lead to blood clotting
D. Is converted to bicarbonate by the liver

22 During a blood transfusion, Mr. R. becomes restless and apprehensive; he complains of chest and lumbar pain. The nurse should immediately:

A. Stop the transfusion
B. Notify the physician
C. Take the patient's vital signs
D. Change the I.V. tubing and filter

23 The physician prescribes cortisone for Mr. R. to take at home after discharge. The nurse should tell the patient to immediately report:

A. Glycosuria
B. Weight gain
C. Mood changes
D. Elevated temperature

SITUATION

J., a 21-year-old African American student who has had sickle cell anemia since early childhood, is admitted to the emergency department (ED) in sickle cell crisis. He says he felt fine until the previous day, when he developed severe diarrhea. He is admitted to the medical unit with orders for bed rest, 50 mg of meperidine (Demerol) I.M. for pain every 3 to 4 hours as needed, and infusion of 1,000 ml of lactated Ringer's solution at 125 ml/hour.

Questions 24 to 28 refer to this situation.

24 When developing J.'s care plan, the nurse should give priority to:

A. Preventing hypostatic pneumonia
B. Relieving pain
C. Preventing skin breakdown
D. Preventing constipation

25 The primary reason for administering lactated Ringer's solution to the patient is to:

A. Replace fluids and dilute sickled cells
B. Reduce blood viscosity, replace electrolytes, and help correct acidity
C. Decrease cellular hydration and replace electrolytes
D. Increase the extracellular compartment's osmolality

26 Despite receiving meperidine (Demerol) every 3 hours, J. is still experiencing diaphoresis and severe pain. A CBC reveals a hemoglobin level of 7 g/dl, a hematocrit of 26%, and a mean corpuscular hemoglobin concentration of 40%. Which therapy will the physician probably order?

A. Packed RBC transfusion
B. Cryoprecipitate transfusion
C. Whole blood transfusion
D. Partial exchange transfusion

27
Which assessment finding would *not* be expected in J.?

A. Splenomegaly
B. Hepatomegaly
C. Jaundice
D. Hematuria

28
The physician orders folic acid (vitamin B₉) therapy for J. to:

A. Correct a deficiency caused by decreased food intake
B. Prevent the development of neurologic problems
C. Correct chronic hemolytic anemia
D. Meet the body's increased demand for folic acid

Within a few days, J. is walking and eating better and has stopped requesting pain medication. The physician orders his discharge and prescribes prednisone (Deltasone), folic acid, and multivitamins.

Questions 29 and 30 continue the situation.

29
Which topic of discussion is the most critical for the nurse to cover during the patient-teaching session before J.'s discharge?

A. Conditions that cause sickle cell crisis
B. The need to wear a medical alert bracelet
C. Adverse effects of steroid therapy
D. The need for regular follow-up examinations and blood tests

30
Because sickle cell anemia causes chronic obstruction of blood to the bones, J. is susceptible to:

A. Ulcers along the medial malleolus
B. Deformities of the metacarpals
C. Necrosis of the hip
D. Multiple fractures

SITUATION

Mr. O., a 55-year-old accountant, is admitted to the ED complaining of increasing episodes of epistaxis, blurred vision, headache, and tinnitus. Examination reveals a blood pressure of 180/100 mm Hg, pitting edema of the legs, and ruddy cyanosis of the face. After reviewing Mr. O.'s family medical history, the physician orders blood tests to assess for polycythemia vera.

Questions 31 to 34 refer to this situation.

31 Which assessment finding is *not* a characteristic clinical manifestation of polycythemia vera?

A. Splemomegaly
B. Plethora
C. Pruritus
D. Elevated temperature (over 100° F [37.8° C])

32 Which nursing intervention would *not* be appropriate for Mr. O.?

A. Restricting fluids to reduce overload
B. Encouraging frequent ambulation
C. Applying extra lotion during skin care
D. Recording the patient's weight and abdominal girth daily

33 While undergoing frequent phlebotomies, Mr. O. should avoid:

A. Taking aspirin
B. Carrying packages
C. Eating highly seasoned food
D. Consuming large amounts of liver and legumes

34 Mr. O.'s drug therapy after discharge is 100 mg of cyclophosphamide (Cytoxin) P.O. daily and 0.5 mg of colchicine (Colsalide) P.O. twice daily. Which type of effect does colchicine have?

A. Anti-inflammatory
B. Analgesic
C. Uricosuric
D. Antipyretic

SITUATION

Mr. H., a 47-year-old janitor with a history of chronic dermatitis, is admitted to the ED in shock from extensive third-degree burns over his chest and arms. The physician orders insertion of an indwelling urinary (Foley) catheter, instillation of lactated Ringer's solution I.V., and wound care using silver sulfadiazine (Silvadene) ointment. Because Mr. H. is bleeding excessively from injection and I.V. sites, the physician orders blood tests to assess for disseminated intravascular coagulation (DIC).

Questions 35 and 36 refer to this situation.

35 Which assessment finding is *not* an expected clinical manifestation of DIC?

A. Petechiae
B. Thrombosis
C. Splenomegaly
D. Acrocyanosis

36 The nurse should alert the physician immediately if assessment reveals:

A. Urine output of 100 ml/hour
B. Epistaxis
C. Chest pain
D. Bleeding gums after brushing teeth

SITUATION

Ms. T., age 25, complains of chronic fatigue, particularly after menstrual periods, which she says sometimes last for 6 days; her sanitary pads often are saturated in 2 hours. After a general practitioner prescribed oral ferrous sulfate (Feosol) therapy, Ms. T. remained fatigued and pale, and tiny bruises appeared on her arms. An internist then referred her to a hematologist, who diagnosed idiopathic thrombocytopenic purpura (ITP) and admitted her to the hospital.

Questions 37 to 39 refer to this situation.

37 Which assessment finding is *not* typical of ITP?

A. Prolonged bleeding
B. Decreased platelet count
C. Increased capillary fragility
D. Prolonged activated partial thromboplastin time

38 The physician orders 60 mg of prednisone P.O. daily, bed rest, and a regular diet for Ms. T. The beneficial effects of prednisone do *not* include:

A. Increased platelet production
B. Increased phagocytic activity in the reticuloendothelial system
C. Suppressed phagocytic activity in the spleen
D. Reduced capillary fragility

39 To minimize the gastric distress associated with oral corticosteroids, the nurse should:

A. Mix prednisone with food
B. Administer the drug before meals
C. Give the drug with an antacid as ordered
D. Give prednisone first when administering with other drugs

Despite daily prednisone therapy, Ms. T.'s platelet count drops. Her prednisone dose is increased to 80 mg daily. During this time, she starts her menses with severe painful menorrhagia.

Questions 40 and 41 continue the situation.

40 Which order should the nurse discuss with the physician before implementation?

A. Taking a platelet count immediately
B. Increasing the daily dosage of prednisone
C. Arranging a gynecologic consultation
D. Administering 600 mg of aspirin every 3 hours as needed

41 Daily platelet counts show a steady increase. When the count reaches 95,000/mm^3, Ms. T. is discharged. The nurse should tell her that long-term prednisone therapy may cause:

A. Hyperglycemia
B. Hypotension
C. Marked weight loss
D. Hypoglycemia

SITUATION

Mr. S., a 24-year-old salesman with classic hemophilia, comes to the clinic because of his concern about transmitting the disease to his children. He has experienced intermittent joint swelling and nosebleeds.

Questions 42 to 44 refer to this situation.

42 Mr. S. suddenly begins to complain of difficulty swallowing. The nurse's first action should be:

A. Auscultating breath sounds
B. Inspecting the oral pharynx
C. Obtaining a tracheostomy set
D. Palpating the thyroid gland

43 Mr. S. seems subdued after a conference with the physician. When the nurse asks why, Mr. S. states that the physician recommended using a commercially prepared antihemophilic factor and that he is worried about contracting acquired immunodeficiency syndrome (AIDS). How should the nurse respond?

A. "For the last few years, all blood donors are tested for AIDS and hepatitis before donating blood"
B. "Only the red blood cells are used in preparing the product"
C. "Donors receive penicillin prophylactically before donating blood"
D. "AIDS is transmitted only by sexual contact"

44 Before discharge, Mr. S. asks the nurse about resuming active participation in sports. The nurse should caution Mr. S. to avoid:

A. Tennis
B. Bowling
C. Golf
D. Football

SITUATION

Mr. L., age 24, is an AIDS patient with a diagnosis of Pneumocystis carinii pneumonia. During 2 weeks of hospitalization with isolation precautions, he has had no visitors.

Questions 45 to 51 refer to this situation.

45 Mr. L.'s strongest feeling at this time is probably:

A. Loss
B. Rejection
C. Ambivalence
D. Anger

46 The worst fear of the patient with AIDS typically is related to:

A. Treatment
B. Disfigurement
C. Self-image
D. Prognosis

47 Human immunodeficiency virus is transmitted in all of the following ways *except:*

A. Through sexual intercourse
B. Through the sharing of drug users' needles
C. To infants of infected mothers either before or during birth
D. Through mosquito and tick bites

48 The patient with AIDS-related complex typically has a history of:

A. Oral candidiasis, molluscum contagiosum, and bullous impetigo
B. Hairy leukoplakia of the tongue and a chronic cough
C. Memory loss, night sweats, and disorientation
D. Severe fatigue, lymphadenopathy, and diarrhea

49 The collapse of the immune response defenses in the AIDS patient stems from which defect?

A. Insufficient amounts of immunoglobulins
B. Overproduction of immature B lymphocytes
C. Reduction in the number and change in the function of CD4 T cells
D. Decreased amounts of tissue macrophage

50 Which type of infection control does an extremely ill hospitalized patient with AIDS require?

A. Respiratory isolation
B. Blood and body fluid precautions
C. Contact isolation
D. Reverse isolation

51 When providing information before Mr. L.'s discharge, the nurse should *not:*

A. Encourage him to use disposable eating and drinking utensils
B. Discuss ways to reduce physical and psychological stress
C. Caution him against sharing razors or toothbrushes with others
D. Advise him to inform his dentist of the condition

SITUATION

Mr. S., age 55, is admitted to the hospital with a diagnosis of chronic lymphocytic leukemia.

Questions 52 to 55 refer to this situation.

52 During routine care, Mr. S. asks the nurse, "How can I be anemic if this disease causes increased white cell production?" The nurse's best response would be that the increased number of white blood cells (WBCs):

A. Crowd out red blood cells
B. Are not responsible for the anemia
C. Use nutrients from other cells
D. Have an abnormally short life span

53 Diagnostic assessment of Mr. S. would probably *not* reveal:

A. A predominance of lymphocytes
B. Leukocytosis with a shift to the left
C. Abnormal blast cells in the bone marrow
D. An elevated thrombocyte count

54 Several days after admission, Mr. S. becomes disoriented and complains of frequent headaches. The nurse's first action should be to:

A. Call the physician
B. Document the patient's status in detail on his chart
C. Prepare oxygen equipment
D. Raise the bed's side rails

55 Which statement about bone marrow transplantation—the treatment of choice for patients under age 40 with leukemia—is *not* correct?

A. The patient is under local anesthesia during the procedure
B. The bone marrow aspirated is mixed with heparin
C. The aspiration site is the posterior or anterior iliac crest
D. The recipient receives cyclophosphamide (Cytoxan) for 4 consecutive days before the procedure

---

SITUATION

Mrs. T., age 53, has been experiencing bone pain, recurrent infections, and abdominal pain for the past 5 years. After ordering a battery of tests, including X-ray studies, the physician diagnoses multiple myeloma.

Questions 56 and 57 refer to this situation.

56 The physician orders administration of melphalan (Alkeran) for Mrs. T. Because this drug causes pancytopenia, the nurse should assess the patient for:

A. Alopecia
B. Skin pigmentation changes
C. Thrombophlebitis
D. Decreased WBC count

57 Nursing care for Mrs. T. should include:

A. Giving 2,000 ml of fluids daily
B. Giving more than 3,000 ml of fluid daily
C. Restricting fluid intake to equal the patient's insensible fluid loss
D. Encouraging increased intake of fluids, particularly milk

SITUATION

Mrs. K., age 59, is admitted to the hospital with a tentative diagnosis of stage III B Hodgkin's disease.

Questions 58 to 60 refer to this situation.

58 Which assessment finding strongly indicates Hodgkin's disease?

A. Night sweats
B. Enlarged lymph nodes
C. Reed-Sternberg cells
D. Hepatomegaly

59 The usual drug therapy for the patient with stage III B Hodgkin's disease is called MOPP. The "O" in MOPP stands for:

A. Prednisone (Orasone)
B. Vincristine (Oncovin)
C. Oxacillin (Bactocill)
D. Oxamniquine (Vansil)

60 Which nursing intervention is most effective in relieving nausea and vomiting associated with MOPP therapy?

A. Administering an antiemetic simultaneously with the drug
B. Encouraging the patient to drink hot liquids, such as coffee or tea
C. Giving an antiemetic 1 to 3 hours before MOPP administration
D. Providing frequent oral hygiene

Answer sheet

	A B C D		A B C D
1	○ ○ ○ ○	31	○ ○ ○ ○
2	○ ○ ○ ○	32	○ ○ ○ ○
3	○ ○ ○ ○	33	○ ○ ○ ○
4	○ ○ ○ ○	34	○ ○ ○ ○
5	○ ○ ○ ○	35	○ ○ ○ ○
6	○ ○ ○ ○	36	○ ○ ○ ○
7	○ ○ ○ ○	37	○ ○ ○ ○
8	○ ○ ○ ○	38	○ ○ ○ ○
9	○ ○ ○ ○	39	○ ○ ○ ○
10	○ ○ ○ ○	40	○ ○ ○ ○
11	○ ○ ○ ○	41	○ ○ ○ ○
12	○ ○ ○ ○	42	○ ○ ○ ○
13	○ ○ ○ ○	43	○ ○ ○ ○
14	○ ○ ○ ○	44	○ ○ ○ ○
15	○ ○ ○ ○	45	○ ○ ○ ○
16	○ ○ ○ ○	46	○ ○ ○ ○
17	○ ○ ○ ○	47	○ ○ ○ ○
18	○ ○ ○ ○	48	○ ○ ○ ○
19	○ ○ ○ ○	49	○ ○ ○ ○
20	○ ○ ○ ○	50	○ ○ ○ ○
21	○ ○ ○ ○	51	○ ○ ○ ○
22	○ ○ ○ ○	52	○ ○ ○ ○
23	○ ○ ○ ○	53	○ ○ ○ ○
24	○ ○ ○ ○	54	○ ○ ○ ○
25	○ ○ ○ ○	55	○ ○ ○ ○
26	○ ○ ○ ○	56	○ ○ ○ ○
27	○ ○ ○ ○	57	○ ○ ○ ○
28	○ ○ ○ ○	58	○ ○ ○ ○
29	○ ○ ○ ○	59	○ ○ ○ ○
30	○ ○ ○ ○	60	○ ○ ○ ○

Answers and rationales

1 Correct answer—**B**

A parasitic infection causes the body to produce large numbers of eosinophils, a type of granulocyte, for phagocytosis—the destruction of particulate matter by leukocytes that engulf and ingest it. Eosinophils also tend to collect in tissue where an allergic reaction has occurred. Monocytes are agranulocytes present in large numbers with long-term chronic infection. Basophils are granulocytes present in large numbers with an allergic reaction; they release histamine in the tissue. Neutrophils, which also are granulocytes, are produced in large numbers with acute inflammation.

2 Correct answer—**A**

Neutrophils, also called polymorphonuclear granulocytes, are the first line of defense when tissue is injured. Eosinophils increase with hypersensitivity (allergic) reactions. Erythrocytes carry oxygen to tissues but do not attack antigens. Platelets are necessary for blood coagulation; they help seal off an open wound but do not attack antigens.

3 Correct answer—**B**

Passive immunity can be transferred through antiserum or gamma globulin (immunoglobulin) injection, which is derived from the sera of those previously immunized or recovering from specific diseases. Natural passive immunity in an infant comes from maternal antibodies transferred across the placental barrier. Natural immunity occurs after having a disease. Active immunity requires the host to produce antibodies.

4 Correct answer—**B**

Antivenoms are passive immunologic products that contain elevated levels of immune globulins which detoxify poisons. Rubella contact resulting in a titer greater than 1:8 confers active immunity. Exposure without developing the disease may also confer active immunity. Measles, mumps, and rubella vaccinations provide active immunity by introducing attenuated (weakened) or dead organisms to the body, stimulating the antibody production.

5 Correct answer—**B**

Administering epinephrine should be the first intervention for anaphylactic shock, which occurs from a hypersensitivity reaction to histamine and histamine-like substances released into the blood;

such reactions cause vasodilation, increased capillary permeability, and contraction of the smooth muscle bronchioles. Airway obstruction may result from laryngeal edema. Epinephrine acts upon the beta₂ receptors, causing bronchodilation. High Fowler's position may be warranted with dyspnea but may not be indicated if the patient is hypotensive. Sodium bicarbonate is not warranted unless high levels of lactic acid are produced with hypoxia. Oxygen therapy usually is necessary but does not correct bronchospasm.

6 Correct answer—D

A tuberculin test that causes induration of 10 mm or more is considered positive, or clinically significant; it indicates exposure to *Mycobacterium tuberculosis.* The body's normal response to antigens is some sign of tissue reaction; it does not mean the patient has allergies. This test screens for tuberculosis but does not confirm the diagnosis.

7 Correct answer—A

B lymphocytes differentiate into plasma cells, which produce immunoglobulins. T lymphocytes control cell-mediated immunity and directly attack antigens through the action of lymphokines. Macrophages process the antigen and present it to the B lymphocyte, which is then stimulated to produce antibodies. Neutrophils do not produce antibodies.

8 Correct answer—C

Cyclophosphamide (Cytoxan) is an immunosuppressive drug used in cancer therapy; because it makes the patient more susceptible to infection, he should avoid people with infections. The patient taking an immunosuppressant should eat cooked vegetables and fruits rather than raw ones, which have organisms on their surfaces. A firm-bristled toothbrush may cause trauma of the gums and buccal mucosa, making them more susceptible to infection; the patient should use a soft-bristled toothbrush instead. Mild lotions and soaps have no adverse effects; the patient should use them to keep the skin clean and dry and to prevent skin breakdown.

9 Correct answer—A

Tophi are sodium urate deposits that develop with gout; they are not seen with systemic lupus erythematosus (SLE). Fever, malaise, and joint, skin, and serous problems are common clinical manifestations of SLE. Other common assessment findings include butterfly rash, arthritis, pleuritis, mild anemia, positive LE cell preparation and antinuclear antibodies titer, and hypocomplementemia.

10 Correct answer—A

Cellulitis is a diffuse inflammatory reaction involving cellular or connective tissue. Cellular death from hypoxia or ischemia is more extreme; the tissue forms eschar—a hard, black outer layer that may be a sign of impending gangrene. A furuncle is a localized cellular response to trauma with purulent exudate. Hyperplasia, a reversible state, is a form of cellular adaptation to injury in which the number of cells in tissue increases.

11 Correct answer—A

Erythrocyte indices, the most reliable diagnostic test for iron deficiency anemia, measure the size and hemoglobin content of erythrocytes, or red blood cells (RBCs). The indices include mean corpuscular volume, mean corpuscular hemoglobin (MCH), and MCH concentration; the results can identify different types of anemia by the cells' size and by hemoglobin concentration in individual cells or a certain volume of cells. The normal MCH is 26 to 32 picograms (pg)/erythrocyte; values less than 26 pg/erythrocyte indicate hemoglobin deficiency (hypochromia) and microcytic cells, which characterize iron deficiency anemia. Total erythrocyte count provides only the number of erythrocytes in a microliter of whole blood; it is used to help compute the erythrocyte indices, but cannot confirm iron deficiency anemia by itself. The hemoglobin test provides the hemoglobin concentration; this test does not indicate the cell's size and fluctuates with both anemia and hydration changes. The hematocrit (HCT) test provides information about the body's hydration state; the HCT level may be decreased with some anemias, but this may also indicate blood loss or a dilutional increase in intravascular volume. HCT levels are more useful for diagnosing polycythemia vera.

12 Correct answer—A

Only about half of the iron will be absorbed; the rest will be eliminated in the feces, turning the patient's stools black or dark green. Iron tablets do not stain teeth; liquid iron may have this effect if not taken through a straw. Iron intake does not affect urine concentration unless iron overload occurs. Iron tablets do not leave a metallic aftertaste in the mouth because the drug is broken down in the stomach and intestine, not the mouth; iron liquid may leave a metallic aftertaste if it is not sufficiently diluted.

13 Correct answer—C

Before the Schilling test, the nurse should instruct the patient to save all but the first urine specimen for the next 24 hours; the urine is examined to evaluate how much vitamin B_{12} is excreted and absorbed. Drinking eight glasses of water would make the test less effective; the patient should drink nothing for 8 to 12 hours before the test. Because the amount of radioactive vitamin B_{12} administered for the test is small, the patient does not need to remain isolated. The first urine specimen—the urine secreted during the night before the radioactive vitamin is administered—should be discarded, but the last one should not.

14 Correct answer—A

Incoordination and weakness of the extremities is a clinical manifestation of pernicious anemia, not folic acid (vitamin B_9) deficiency anemia. A sore, beefy tongue (caused by insufficient hydrochloric acid in the stomach and possibly by coexisting thiamine deficiency) and nausea and anorexia are common with most anemias. Tachycardia also is common in all anemias in varying degrees, depending on the anemia's severity.

15 Correct answer—D

The nurse should not discontinue oxygen without the physician's order; a nasal cannula does not interfere with eating and need not be removed for meals. The nurse should change the cannula according to institutional policy because nasal secretions adhere to the cannula prongs; these secretions may cause infection. Humidifying the oxygen is necessary because prolonged exposure of the mucous membranes to high flow rates of oxygen without humidification causes irritation and damage. The nurse should assess for signs of hypoxia, which may indicate cannula prong dislodgment or worsening of the patient's condition; if signs of hypoxia appear, arterial blood gas levels should be assessed immediately.

16 Correct answer—C

Liver and asparagus are both rich sources of folic acid. Besides organ meats and green, leafy vegetables, good sources of folic acid include kidney beans, wheat germ, and nuts. Chicken and fish are not particularly rich sources of folic acid; eggs, root vegetables, most fruits, and milk are also poor sources.

17 Correct answer—B

The patient's prolonged bleeding time and other possible hematologic problems increase his risk of developing a hematoma, a localized collection of extravasated blood in the tissue; the nurse should
apply ice packs to the aspiration site because cold has a vasocon-
stricting effect on blood vessels. Applying extra pressure to the site
for 5 to 10 minutes also helps constrict blood vessels. Having the patient lie on the aspiration site will not prevent hematoma formation
and may cause discomfort. The needle puncture should require
only a small adhesive bandage; this allows the nurse to see if a hematoma is developing but does not help prevent it. Povidone-iodine
solution does not help prevent hematoma formation; it is used to
clean the aspiration site before the procedure to prevent infection.

18 Correct answer—C

The nurse should try to prevent infection. Neutropenia—a decrease
in the number of white blood cells—is the main cause of the granu-
locytic state, compromising phagocytosis and increasing the risk of
infection. Hemorrhages, bruises, and fatigue are not related to granulocytopenia. Hemorrhage and bruising result from a low platelet
count and prolonged bleeding time; fatigue results from the reduction in the number of RBCs.

19 Correct answer—D

The plasma of type AB blood does not contain anti-A or anti-B agglutinins. The four major blood types (A, B, AB, and O) are based on
the agglutinogens (antigens) present in the RBCs. Individuals have
acquired or inherited antibodies against agglutinogens called agglutinins. With type AB blood, the RBCs have A and B agglutinogens
and the plasma is free of anti-A and anti-B agglutinins; otherwise,
the individual's own RBCs would be attacked, causing hemolytic reactions. Individuals with type AB blood are called universal blood recipients because with no anti-A or anti-B agglutinins in their plasma,
they can receive any type of blood without hemolytic reaction.

20 Correct answer—A

The most critical nursing action when administering blood products
is ensuring that the correct recipient receives the correct blood
product; administration of the wrong blood product can cause potentially fatal physiologic reactions. Explaining the procedure to the patient, assessing for fluid overload, and using the appropriate filter
are important nursing actions but not as critical as verifying the recipient and the blood product.

21 Correct answer—C

Lactated Ringer's solution contains calcium, which may lead to blood clotting if blood is administered. Administering dextrose, not lactated Ringer's solution, before blood causes hemolysis of the RBCs. Lactated Ringer's solution is isotonic, with an osmolality of 272 mOsm/liter; normal serum osmolality is 275 to 300 mOsm/liter. Lactate is converted to bicarbonate by the liver, but this is not related to blood transfusion and is not a contraindication.

22 Correct answer—A

Restlessness, apprehension, and complaints of chest and lumbar pain during blood transfusion indicate a hemolytic reaction; the nurse should immediately stop the transfusion to prevent further harmful and even fatal effects. After stopping the transfusion, the nurse should take the patient's vital signs (which provide parameters for intervention) and call the physician. The nurse should keep the I.V. line in place and infuse normal saline solution to keep the vein open.

23 Correct answer—D

The patient should immediately report an elevated temperature, which indicates a breakdown in immune response; this is critical because granulocytopenia already has compromised the patient's immune response. Cortisone is a glucocorticoid, a hormone produced by the adrenal cortex. Its effects include inhibiting inflammation; suppressing the immune response; increasing blood coagulability, resistance to stress, and retention of sodium and water; and altering nutritional status and energy level. Glycosuria and weight gain may result from prolonged use of steroids, not glucocorticoids. Mood changes are common with glucocorticoid use, but they are not dangerous or life-threatening.

24 Correct answer—B

Because the patient was admitted in sickle cell crisis, which causes intense pain, the nurse's immediate priority is relieving pain. Pain causes excessive perspiration, dehydrating the patient and worsening the crisis. The other nursing goals are important but do not require the immediate attention pain relief does; their aim is to prevent complications of prolonged bed rest. Hypostatic pneumonia may result from sluggish GI peristalsis and the pooling of secretions in the lungs; skin breakdown may result from immobility and extra pressure on the skin; and constipation may result from lack of activity, sluggish peristalsis, and changes in diet and fluid intake.

25 Correct answer—B

Lactated Ringer's solution reduces blood viscosity, replaces electrolytes, and helps correct acidity (through the conversion of lactate to bicarbonate by the liver). In a sickle cell crisis, hypoxia, stress, infection, or dehydration (as from severe diarrhea) causes RBCs to stiffen and become sickle-shaped, increasing blood viscosity and occluding capillaries; this increases hypoxia and leads to anaerobic metabolism, producing lactic and pyruvic acid. The increased viscosity reduces the circulatory rate and decreases blood volume to the kidneys. The patient needs large volumes of fluids to decrease sickling and replace fluids and electrolytes lost from fever and diaphoresis, but he also needs something to reverse the acidity; lactated Ringer's solution does all these things. Decreasing cellular hydration would probably cause sickling, not correct it. Lactated Ringer's solution, which is isotonic, would not change the osmolality of the extracellular compartment.

26 Correct answer—D

Partial exchange transfusion, the preferred treatment method, removes some of the sickled cells and replaces them with healthy, nonsickled cells. The removal of some of the sickled cells decreases blood viscosity, increasing tissue oxygenation and decreasing pain. Most patients require several exchange transfusions. Giving packed RBCs without removing sickled cells would be the least effective treatment method because the excess RBCs would cause the spleen to destroy both sickle cells and healthy cells; the patient's condition would not improve and might even worsen. Cryoprecipitate, a plasma derivative containing some clotting factors but no platelets, would not help this patient because sickle cell crisis increases blood viscosity, not the risk of excessive bleeding. Because of the patient's long-standing history of sickle cell anemia, some heart enlargement probably is present; whole blood transfusion is contraindicated because it may result in cardiac overload.

27 Correct answer—A

Splenomegaly would not be an expected assessment finding. Because the patient has had sickle cell anemia since childhood, autosplenectomy—shrinkage of the spleen from repeated infarction and fibrosis—is an expected finding. Jaundice and hepatomegaly are typical findings in the patient with long-standing sickle cell anemia because of accelerated bilirubin production from RBC destruction. Hematuria is a common result of repeated occlusion and infarction, which cause renal papillary necrosis.

28 Correct answer—C

Sickle cell anemia causes accelerated destruction of RBCs, resulting in chronic hemolytic anemia; because folic acid (vitamin B_9) is necessary for RBC maturation, folic acid therapy should allow RBCs to mature faster than they are destroyed, correcting hemolytic anemia. Decreased food intake would not cause folic acid deficiency unless it involved decreased intake of green, leafy vegetables and other rich sources of folic acid. Vitamin B_{12}, not folic acid, controls central nervous system function; folic acid therapy would not prevent the development of neurologic problems. Because the patient is not going through an increased growth spurt, the body would not have an increased demand for folic acid.

29 Correct answer—A

The patient apparently does not fully understand the causes of sickle cell crisis; otherwise, he would have sought medical attention to stop his diarrhea, a condition that causes fluid loss, dehydration, and subsequent sickling. The need to wear a medical alert bracelet, the adverse effects of steroid therapy, and the need for follow-up medical examinations and blood tests are also important, but they are not as critical as the causes of sickle cell crisis.

30 Correct answer—C

In adults with sickle cell anemia, obstruction of a major artery may lead to avascular necrosis of the femoral head or of the humerus. Some patients are placed on bed rest and later use crutches to relieve the pressure on these weight-bearing joints, but necrosis continues even with these measures; eventually, patients require a total joint replacement. Ulcers along the medial malleolus are caused by occlusion of blood vessels, most often resulting from external pressure. Deformities of the metacarpals are more common in young children, who sometimes develop a condition called hand-foot syndrome, or sickle cell dactylitis. Multiple fractures are not associated with obstruction of blood to the bones in sickle cell anemia.

31 Correct answer—D

Elevated temperature is not a characteristic clinical manifestation of polycythemia vera. This disorder is characterized by unrestrained erythrocyte production as well as excessive production of myelocytes and platelets; it causes increased blood viscosity, increased total blood volume (up to three times the normal volume), and severe congestion of all tissues and organs. Splenomegaly is a clinical manifestation of polycythemia vera; its exact cause is unknown, but it may result from extramedullary erythropoiesis and proliferation of the endoplasmic reticulum. Plethora—an excessive accumulation of blood—causes the ruddy cyanosis of the face, nose, ears, and lips typically seen in light-skinned patients with polycythemia vera. Histamine release by granulocytes causes pruritus in about 40% of patients with the disorder. Other clinical manifestations include visual disturbances, ecchymosis, thrombosis, and hemorrhage.

32 Correct answer—A

Restricting fluids is inappropriate; this would make the patient's thick, sluggish blood even more viscous, increasing the risk of thrombus formation. Unless contraindicated, the nurse should increase the patient's fluid intake, which helps dilute the blood and rid the body of excess uric acid via the kidneys. Frequent ambulation stimulates skeletal muscle contraction, improving venous return. Applying extra lotion during skin care is recommended because dry skin stimulates itching. Recording weight and abdominal girth helps the nurse assess for internal bleeding.

33 Correct answer—D

Organ meats, such as liver, and legumes, such as beans and peas, are high in iron; a high iron intake increases erythrocyte production, counteracting the effects of phlebotomies. Aspirin may be beneficial because it interferes with platelet aggregation, decreasing the risk of thrombosis. Unless the patient has an arteriovenous shunt, carrying packages is not contraindicated. Avoiding highly seasoned food is not necessary unless the patient has a peptic ulcer, which commonly accompanies polycythemia vera.

34 Correct answer—A

Colchicine (Colsalide) has an anti-inflammatory effect. Excessive cellular proliferation increases degradation of nucleoprotein; this increases uric acid levels, causing gout symptoms. Colchicine reduces the body's response to inflammation from urate crystals deposited in the joints. The reduced inflammation indirectly decreases pain; however, colchicine does not have a direct analgesic, uricosuric, or antipyretic effect.

35 Correct answer—C

Splenomegaly rarely occurs with DIC; the spleen usually enlarges in response to increased activity only over a prolonged period, and DIC typically has an acute onset. Common clinical manifestations of DIC, which relate directly to impaired coagulation, include petechiae, thrombosis, acrocyanosis (Raynaud's sign), purpura, and ecchymosis.

36 Correct answer—C

Because of generalized microthrombi formation, embolism is a constant threat; the nurse should alert the physician immediately if assessment reveals chest pain, which may indicate a pulmonary embolus. A urine output over 30 ml/hour is considered adequate. A single episode of epistaxis, which may result from various causes, does not require the physician's immediate attention, but it should be noted. Bleeding gums after brushing teeth may indicate a coagulation problem, but it is not a critical sign of excessive bleeding.

37 Correct answer—D

Prolonged activated partial thromboplastin time is not a typical assessment finding with idiopathic thrombocytopenic purpura (ITP). Thrombocytopenia refers to a platelet count below 100,000/mm³, which is caused by premature platelet destruction. Normally, platelets survive 8 to 10 days; with thrombocytopenia, the survival rate is 2 to 3 days. Bone marrow aspiration reveals normal or increased megakaryocytes (precursors to platelets). Platelets form temporary clots, release incomplete thromboplastin, and maintain capillary integrity; they help close openings in capillary walls and improve clot strength and retraction. Because of the low platelet count, bleeding is prolonged, capillary fragility is increased, and megakaryocytes are normal or increased. Platelets alone do not control bleeding; other coagulation factors from the intrinsic and extrinsic systems are necessary for homeostasis. Because these factors are intact, coagulation time is not affected; the activated partial thromboplastin time is normal.

38 Correct answer—B

Prednisone does not increase the phagocytic action in the reticuloendothelial system; this would not be a beneficial effect for treating ITP. The drug causes increased platelet production, reduced capillary fragility, and suppressed phagocytosis within parts of the reticuloendothelial system, such as the spleen. The exact mechanism by which prednisone mediates these actions is unknown.

39 Correct answer—C

Oral corticosteroids, such as prednisone, cause gastric distress by increasing gastric secretions, which causes bleeding and peptic ulceration. To prevent this, the nurse should give the drug with an antacid. If the physician does not order an antacid, the nurse should give the drug after meals; giving steroids on an empty stomach increases GI distress because the gastric mucosa has no protective coating. Administering steroids first with multiple drug therapy has no effect unless all are given after meals or with an antacid. Mixing prednisone with food may cause the patient to develop a dislike for the particular food.

40 Correct answer—D

Aspirin is contraindicated in thrombocytopenia because it interferes with platelet aggregation and increases the risk of excessive bleeding. Because prednisone increases platelet production, a platelet count helps determine the drug's effectiveness on extreme menorrhagia. The physician probably would increase the prednisone dosage if the platelet count results were still low. Because the patient is in pain, the physician may suspect a coexisting condition, such as endometriosis; a gynecologic consultation is appropriate.

41 Correct answer—A

Prednisone is a synthetic steroid containing glucocorticoid hormones, which control gluconeogenesis (glucose formation from amino acids and fats in the liver). Therefore, prednisone use increases glucose levels and long-term therapy may cause hyperglycemia, not hypoglycemia. Steroids typically cause fluid retention, resulting in weight gain, fluid and electrolyte imbalances, and possible hypertension.

42 Correct answer—C

The nurse's first action should be obtaining a tracheostomy set because difficulty in swallowing may indicate bleeding into subcutaneous tissue. The Factor VIII deficiency associated with classic hemophilia (hemophilia A) causes severe uncontrolled bleeding in the joints (hemarthrosis), GI tract, subcutaneous tissue, and urinary system; bleeding may occur several hours after trauma, causing swelling and pressure on nerve endings. Auscultating breath sounds is inappropriate because it does not provide information about the patient's complaint. Inspecting the pharynx would not provide much information, and the nurse's first priority when a patient with hemophilia has difficulty swallowing is to ensure a patent airway. Palpation of the thyroid may reveal an increase in size, but thyroid enlargement would not cause a sudden difficulty in swallowing.

43 Correct answer—A

Since 1985, hospitals and blood centers have tested blood donors for acquired immunodeficiency syndrome (AIDS); they have tested for various forms of hepatitis for more than 10 years. The commercially prepared product is prepared from pooled donor plasma, not red blood cells (RBCs); clotting factors, particularly the antihemophilic globulin, are found in the plasma. Penicillin does not destroy the viruses and microorganisms that cause AIDS and hepatitis; prophylactic use would not prevent their transmission. Besides sexual contact, AIDS is transmitted through exposure to contaminated blood products.

44 Correct answer—D

Individuals with hemophilia should avoid contact sports, such as football, to prevent bruising and uncontrolled bleeding from the inevitable body contact and trauma. Tennis, bowling, and golf are appropriate sports because they involve no body contact.

45 Correct answer—B

The AIDS patient commonly feels isolated and rejected by friends and stigmatized by the disease. The patient experiences grief and loss; ambivalent feelings toward family, friends, and lovers; and anger at contracting an illness, particularly one so devastating. However, rejection would probably be the patient's strongest feeling in this situation because he has had no visitors.

46 Correct answer—D

The high mortality rate of AIDS creates tremendous fear and depression in patients. They usually have some anxiety related to treatments and concern related to disfigurement and self-image, but the poor prognosis creates the worst fear.

47 Correct answer—D

No evidence suggests that human immunodeficiency virus (HIV) is transmitted through insect bites. The virus is difficult to transmit; exposure requires close contact with the blood or body fluids of an infected person. AIDS is predominantly a sexually transmitted disease; semen and vaginal fluid carry the virus and can enter the body through the vagina, penis, rectum, or mouth. Because needles and syringes of drug abusers are usually not sterilized between use and because many share their needles, the small amount of blood trapped in the drug paraphernalia can transmit the virus. Infected pregnant women have one chance in two of delivering a child with AIDS.

48 Correct answer—**D**

Although a patient with HIV infection may experience no ill effects, the history of a patient with AIDS-related complex typically includes severe fatigue, lymphadenopathy, bouts of diarrhea, malaise, weight loss, night sweats, oral thrush, or several of these disorders. Oral candidiasis, molluscum contagiosum, bullous impetigo, and memory loss by themselves do not necessarily imply HIV infection. Hairy leukoplakia indicates full-blown AIDS.

49 Correct answer—**C**

The AIDS patient commonly has a striking depletion of the CD4 T cells normally found in the blood, lymph nodes, spleen, and other tissues. These cells are lymphocytes, the white blood cells (WBCs) central to immune response. Without CD4 T cells, the B lymphocytes cannot produce enough antibodies (immunoglobulins) to combat the AIDS virus. AIDS does not cause overproduction of immature B lymphocytes. There is no test that measures the amount of tissue macrophage.

50 Correct answer—**B**

The patient with AIDS requires blood and body fluid precautions because HIV is found in the blood and body fluids of infected persons. Therefore, health care providers wear gloves and gowns to prevent contamination with blood, feces, urine, bronchial secretions, or other body fluids. Because HIV is not transmitted by droplet inspiration or by casual contact, respiratory isolation and contact isolation are inappropriate. Reverse isolation, which protects the patient against infection from caregivers and visitors, is unnecessary.

51 Correct answer—**A**

Because AIDS is spread only by contact with an infected person's blood or body fluids, the patient can share utensils if they are washed with detergent and hot water. Discussing ways to reduce stress is appropriate because some experts have noticed sudden deterioration in AIDS patients when confronting excessive physical or psychological stress. Because razors and toothbrushes may have blood or body secretions remaining even after cleaning, the patient should not share them with anyone. Dental care requires contact with oral secretions; the dentist should be told the patient has AIDS to take adequate precautions.

52 Correct answer—A

Uncontrolled proliferation of granulocytes and monocytes causes leukemia, in which WBCs are produced at a rapid rate, crowding out RBCs. This reduces the amount of oxygen-transporting hemoglobin, resulting in anemia. The WBCs do not use nutrients from other cells or have an abnormally short life span.

53 Correct answer—D

Assessment of the patient with leukemia typically reveals thrombocytopenia, rather than an elevated thrombocyte count; with leukemia, an increased number of immature WBCs are produced, crowding out platelets and RBCs. Another common clinical manifestation of leukemia is an increased WBC count with increased release of band (immature) cells by the bone marrow—leukocytosis with a shift to the left. Blast cells, which are precursors of WBCs, accumulate in the bone marrow with leukemia.

54 Correct answer—D

Leukemia causes disorientation and headaches in the patient through WBC infiltration of the central nervous system (CNS); the nurse should raise the bed's side rails to prevent falls. The nurse should document the assessment information after taking action to prevent injury. Administering oxygen will not remove WBCs from the CNS. The nurse should notify the physician of the patient's condition change *after* ensuring his safety.

55 Correct answer—A

The patient is under general or spinal anesthesia during bone marrow transplantation. The procedure involves the aspiration of approximately 600 ml of bone marrow from the iliac crest; the marrow is mixed with heparin or frozen until given intravenously to the recipient. Recipients are "primed" to prevent rejection by receiving cyclophosphasmide (Cytoxan) for 4 days before the transplant. The drug's exact action is unknown; it has been found to have a pronounced immunosuppressive effect.

56 Correct answer—D

Pancytopenia refers to depression in all the blood's cellular elements; the patient on melphalan (Alkeran) therapy would probably have a reduced WBC count. Skin pigmentation is governed by melanocytes, which are controlled by the pituitary gland; because melphalan affects bone marrow production of blood cells, the drug would cause skin pigmentation changes. Temporary alopecia and mild thrombophlebitis at the infusion site are adverse effects of melphalen therapy, but they are not related to pancytopenia.

57 Correct answer—B

The daily fluid intake of the patient with multiple myeloma should be 3,000 to 4,000 ml. Multiple myelomas cause bone destruction and high calcium levels in the bloodstream, and excess plasma cells produce high globulin levels; a high fluid intake helps dilute the calcium overload and prevent protein from precipitating in the renal tubules. Restricting fluids would increase the risk of renal stones. Milk would increase the patient's blood calcium level, possibly contributing to calcium excretion in the urine.

58 Correct answer—C

Reed-Sternberg cells proliferate in the patient with Hodgkin's disease, replacing other cellular elements found in the lymph nodes. Night sweats and enlarged lymph nodes occur with Hodgkin's disease, but they may be caused by other diseases. Hepatomegaly occurs with other conditions, such as cirrhosis, but not with Hodgkin's disease.

59 Correct answer—B

The "O" in MOPP stands for vincristine (Oncovin). The patient with stage III B Hodgkin's disease receives a cyclic drug combination of mechlorethamine (Mustargen), vincristine (Oncovin), procarbazine (Matulane), and prednisone (Orasone); these drugs are given for 14 days, with 14 days' rest between cycles. Oxacillin (Bactocill) is an antibiotic, and oxamniquine (Vansil) is an anthelmintic; neither is part of the drug therapy for Hodgkin's disease.

60 Correct answer—C

The best intervention for relieving nausea and vomiting from MOPP therapy is to administer an antiemetic 1 to 3 hours before starting therapy; this gives the antiemetic time to take effect. An antiemetic administered simultaneously with MOPP therapy may not be as effective. The patient should not drink hot liquids; they appear to contribute to nausea. Frequent oral hygiene may reduce stomatitis, but it does not relieve nausea.

CHAPTER 9

Comprehensive Examination

Questions

1 Which nursing action most effectively reduces postoperative wound infection?

A. Giving an antibiotic I.V. 24 hours postoperatively
B. Not washing the patient's hair the evening before surgery
C. Telling the patient not to shower the day of surgery
D. Shaving the incision site in the operating room

2 A patient should not have any food or drink for at least 8 hours before surgery to:

A. Promote nutritional state
B. Reduce the possibility of aspiration while anesthetized
C. Prevent paralytic ileus
D. Promote the blood supply to the surgical site

3 I.V. fluid intake typically exceeds urine output for 48 to 72 hours postoperatively. Which hormone, secreted during the stress response, is responsible for this?

A. Growth hormone
B. Prolactin
C. Antidiuretic hormone
D. Insulin

4 Mrs. R., age 64, is brought into the emergency department (ED) with a history of loss of appetite and weight loss as well as polydipsia and polyuria. The nurse notes that the patient seems somewhat confused or disoriented and obtains a history from her son. Laboratory values reveal a blood glucose level of 900 mg/dl; serum osmolality of 400 mOsm/kg; absence of plasma ketones; and blood urea nitrogen level of 90 mg/dl. These assessment findings most likely indicate:

A. Hypoglycemic coma
B. Insulin shock
C. Diabetic ketoacidosis
D. Hyperosmolar nonketotic syndrome

5 Mrs. Y., a 35-year-old woman with Type I diabetes mellitus, is admitted to the hospital for I.V. antibiotic therapy for her foot ulcer. She complains of headache, nausea, and abdominal cramps. Her breath has a fruity odor, and her respiratory rate is 30 breaths/minute. Fingerstick reveals a blood glucose level of 398 mg/dl. The nurse should expect the physician to order:

A. Dextrose 5% in water through a wide-open I.V. line
B. Regular insulin and normal saline solution I.V.
C. 20 units of isophane insulin suspension (NPH) and increased fluid intake
D. Aerobic exercises for the patient, to help lower her blood glucose level

6 The best way to evaluate long-term diabetes control is to monitor:

A. Home blood glucose levels
B. Urine tests
C. The fasting blood glucose level
D. The glycosylated hemoglobin (hemoglobin A_{1C}) level

7 Mr. F., a 52-year-old Type II diabetic admitted for control of his diabetes, complains about impotence. The nurse's best response would be:

A. "Have the physician check your testosterone level"
B. "You're probably having a problem with the nerves that cause erection; this may improve with better diabetic control"
C. "You should confine sexual activity to the morning, when you are more rested"
D. "This is probably not related to your diabetes"

8 During the nurse's evening rounds, she finds Mr. G., a Type I diabetic patient, unconscious. The best nursing action would be to:

A. Administer insulin I.V. immediately
B. Give 25 to 50 ml of dextrose 50% by slow I.V. push
C. Start cardiopulmonary resuscitation immediately
D. Administer normal saline solution I.V. and notify the physician immediately

9 Cardiac output refers to:

A. The amount of tension the ventricle must develop during contraction to eject blood from the left ventricle into the aorta
B. The amount of blood ejected by the left ventricle into the aorta per beat
C. The amount of blood ejected by the left ventricle necessary to adequately perfuse the body
D. The amount of blood ejected from the left ventricle into the aorta per minute

10 The PR interval on an electrocardiogram (ECG) corresponds to the period of:

A. Ventricular depolarization
B. Atrial depolarization
C. Impulse conduction between the sinoatrial node and the ventricular musculature
D. Impulse conduction between the atrioventricular node and the ventricular septum

11 An arrhythmia that appears near the peak or deflection of T waves on the ECG is called:

A. The R-on-T phenomenon
B. Premature atrial contractions
C. Junctional rhythm
D. Idioventricular rhythm

12 Which techniques should the nurse teach a patient with bilateral left hemianopia?

A. Scanning techniques
B. Rehabilitation techniques for the right side of his body
C. The proper use of frosted glasses for his left eye
D. Ocular exercises to strengthen the eye muscle to move toward the left

13 Mr. P., a 49-year-old patient recovering from a cerebrovascular accident, has no problems swallowing or eating but cannot tell the nurse what he wants; he gestures toward his bedside stand and waves his arms. This condition is called:

A. Apraxia
B. Aphasia
C. Dysarthria
D. Agnosia

14 Which nursing observation would indicate that peritoneal dialysis has achieved its desired therapeutic effect?

A. The volume of the outflow dialysate equals the volume of the inflow dialysate
B. The patient weighs less than before dialysis
C. Respirations are moist and regular
D. Redness appears on skin near the catheter

15 Peritonitis is a common complication of peritoneal dialysis. Which assessment finding is considered a manifestation of peritonitis?

A. Cloudiness of the drained dialysate
B. Slow outflow rate
C. Redness of the skin around the catheter
D. Difficulty breathing

16 When caring for a patient who has an arteriovenous graft in the left arm, the nurse should *not:*

A. Take all blood pressures in the right arm
B. Infuse I.V. solutions in the left arm above the graft
C. Position the patient on the right side
D. Instruct the patient to exercise the left arm by squeezing a small rubber ball

17 Which information best helps the nurse evaluate the effects of dialysis on a patient?

A. Blood pressure and weight measurements before and after dialysis
B. Daily hemoglobin and hematocrit test results
C. The patient's continuing complaint of dry mouth
D. Inspection of the patient's extremities before and after dialysis

18 When a patient experiences a seizure, the nurse's first action should be to:

A. Pad the bed's side rails
B. Maintain the patient's airway
C. Assess the patient's level of consciousness
D. Provide privacy for the patient

19 Postoperative nursing assessment following temporal lobectomy for uncontrolled seizures should focus specifically on the patient's:

A. Ability to speak
B. Motor function
C. Regulation of body temperature
D. Ability to think abstractly

20 The nurse should assess a patient's nutritional status and nitrogen balance before surgery because:

A. A positive nitrogen balance may adversely affect wound healing
B. Hypoproteinemia is associated with an increased risk of wound infection
C. The patient should be at optimum weight to decrease the risk of infection
D. Excess weight adversely affects wound healing

21 How is malnutrition in postoperative patients linked to infection?

A. Neutrophil levels are diminished postoperatively because of malnutrition
B. Faulty sterile technique increases the risk of infection
C. Adequate dietary intake always prevents postoperative infection
D. Granulocyte activation is increased

22 Mrs. M., age 45, has undergone an abdominal hysterectomy. Three hours later, postoperative assessment reveals a blood pressure of 80/50 mm Hg, temperature of 98.1° F (36.7° C), pulse rate of 130 beats/minute, and pale, cold, clammy skin. These findings indicate:

A. Atelectasis
B. Hypovolemic shock
C. Residual effect of anesthesia
D. Wound infection

23 Which nursing intervention is most appropriate for a myasthenia gravis patient who has difficulty swallowing?

A. Decreasing fluids to 1,000 ml daily and elevating the head of the bed 45 degrees
B. Administering anticholinesterase drugs after meals as ordered and providing only lukewarm foods
C. Providing milk products and having the patient use a straw while drinking
D. Giving the main meal early in the day and providing soft foods that do not require much chewing

24 A patient taking phenytoin (Dilantin) for treatment of trigeminal neuralgia should report which adverse effect to her physician immediately?

A. Easy bruising
B. Decreased facial pain
C. Dry mouth
D. Improved sleeping

25 Which nursing action would be most helpful before a patient with trigeminal neuralgia is discharged?

A. Encouraging the patient to use narcotic pain medications at home, especially before activity
B. Encouraging the patient to participate in an aerobics class at least three times a week
C. Encouraging the patient to eat three large, well-balanced meals a day
D. Helping the patient identify pain trigger zones and ways to prevent pain episodes

26 Mr. P., a 28-year-old man with acquired immunodeficiency syndrome (AIDS), is admitted to the ED with a fever of 102.8° F (39.3° C) and shortness of breath. The physician orders a complete blood count (CBC) with a differential smear. Which special precautions should the nurse take during the phlebotomy?

A. Completing the laboratory requisition for a CBC
B. Antiseptic cleaning of the nurse's hands
C. Wearing gloves and carefully disposing of the needles
D. Aspirating blood without introducing air into the bloodstream

27 Which topic of discussion is most critical when the nurse prepares an AIDS patient for discharge?

A. Transmission methods of the virus
B. The availability of emergency care
C. Signs and symptoms of phlebitis
D. The historic development of AIDS

28 Death from AIDS occurs because of:

A. Overwhelming opportunistic infection
B. Increased killer T cell levels
C. An anaphylactic reaction to antibiotics
D. Malabsorption syndrome

29 When caring for a patient with Parkinson's disease, the nurse should never administer levodopa with:

A. Carbidopa
B. Monoamine oxidase inhibitors
C. Anticholinergic drugs
D. Trihexyphenidyl (Artane)

30 Which assessment finding is *not* associated with increased intracranial pressure?

A. Space-occupying masses
B. Cerebral edema
C. Hydrocephalus
D. Pulmonary edema

31 Which assessment finding does *not* call for endotracheal intubation and mechanical ventilatory support in a patient in respiratory failure?

A. Respiratory rate above 24 breaths/minute
B. Vital capacity lower than 15 ml/kg of body weight
C. Negative inspiratory force less than 25 cm H_2O
D. Arterial hypoxemia and hypercapnia

32 A patient with a long history of smoking, coughing, and sputum production is brought to the ED in respiratory distress. Arterial blood gas (ABG) analysis at admission reveals a pH of 7.20, a partial pressure of carbon dioxide in arterial blood ($Paco_2$) of 75 mm Hg, and a bicarbonate (HCO_3^-) level of 34 mEq/liter. After endotracheal intubation, the patient is placed on a mechanical ventilator. To prudently reduce the $Paco_2$, the nurse should:

A. Ventilate vigorously to bring the $Paco_2$ to 40 mm Hg within 10 minutes
B. Ventilate with low tidal volumes and maintain the $Paco_2$ at 70 mm Hg
C. Ventilate with adequate rate and tidal volume to lower the $Paco_2$ slowly
D. Hyperventilate the patient and administer sodium bicarbonate I.V.

33 A patient with no history of lung disease is given 40% oxygen via Venturi mask. ABG measurements reveal a pH of 7.20, a $PaCO_2$ of 80 mm Hg, and a partial pressure of oxygen in arterial blood (PaO_2) of 65 mm Hg. If the patient becomes drowsy, obtunded, and unable to expectorate, the nurse should:

A. Decrease the fraction of inspired oxygen to 35%
B. Give intermittent positive-pressure breathing treatments
C. Prepare for endotracheal intubation and mechanical ventilation
D. Provide vigorous chest physiotherapy and postural drainage

34 ABG analysis in Mr. Q., a patient breathing room air, reveals a pH of 7.19, a $PaCO_2$ of 42 mm Hg, an HCO_3^- level of 15.7 mEq/liter, and a PaO_2 of 40 mm Hg. The patient has:

A. Metabolic acidosis
B. Compensated metabolic acidosis
C. Respiratory acidosis
D. Metabolic alkalosis

35 During the first hour after a partial thyroidectomy, the nurse should assess for:

A. Aphonia
B. Hoarseness and elevated blood pressure
C. Hypothermia
D. Pneumonia

36 Which assessment finding after thyroid surgery indicates hypocalcemia?

A. Change in level of consciousness
B. Generalized tonic-clonic seizures
C. Nausea and vomiting
D. Muscle tremors

37 Mrs. U., age 30, is admitted to the clinic complaining of intermittently cold, pale, painful hands during summer and winter. The nurse should suspect:

A. Raynaud's syndrome
B. Diabetic angiopathy
C. Venous insufficiency
D. Osteoarthritis

SITUATION

Mr. J., a 55-year-old car salesman, is admitted to the ED because of respiratory distress. He is overweight and has a history of smoking three packs of cigarettes daily for the last 30 years. Physical examination confirms acute respiratory distress. Vital signs reveal a temperature of 101.2° F (38.4° C), a pulse rate of 136 beats/minute, a respiratory rate of 36 breaths/minute, and a blood pressure of 170/92 mm Hg. The patient sits upright, using his accessory muscles for breathing; his skin is reddish blue, and he is perspiring heavily. Auscultation of the chest reveals marked expiratory and inspiratory wheezing. Mr. J. is admitted to the hospital with a diagnosis of chronic obstructive pulmonary disease (COPD).

Questions 38 to 42 refer to this situation.

---

38 The physician orders ABG analysis before oxygen administration begins. The results reveal a pH of 7.25, a $PaCO_2$ of 50 mm Hg, a PaO_2 of 55 mm Hg, and an HCO_3^- level of 25 mEq/liter. These results indicate:

A. Respiratory alkalosis
B. Respiratory acidosis
C. Metabolic alkalosis
D. Metabolic acidosis

---

39 Which assessment findings are *not* characteristic clinical manifestations of COPD?

A. Dyspnea, especially upon exertion
B. Intermittent cough with thick bronchial secretions
C. Flattened diaphragm and increased anteroposterior chest diameter (barrel chest)
D. Anemia and pulmonary hypotension

---

40 The physician orders nasal oxygen for Mr. J. at 2 liters/minute. Which assessment finding should the nurse immediately report to the physician after oxygen therapy begins?

A. Negative Homans' sign
B. Negative Babinski's sign
C. Eupnea
D. Carbon dioxide narcosis

41 Which pharmacologic agent would *not* be used to treat COPD?

A. Bronchodilators
B. Corticosteroids
C. Depressants
D. Aerosols

42 The most critical topic of discussion during Mr. J.'s discharge teaching is:

A. Fluid restriction
B. Pursed-lip expiratory breathing
C. Adequate rest and sleeping in the supine position
D. The need to perform all of his activities at one time

SITUATION

Mr. S., age 42, is admitted to the hospital with pancreatitis. Five months ago, he was hospitalized with the same diagnosis. He has lost 20 lb and has a yellow complexion. He informs the nurse that his urine is dark and that he has been vomiting frequently.

Questions 43 to 47 refer to this situation.

43 Which type of pain is Mr. S. most likely to have?

A. Abdominal pain radiating to his back that is unrelieved by food or antacids
B. Right lower quadrant pain with rebound tenderness
C. Severe abdominal distention and pain with associated bloody diarrhea
D. Indigestion and right upper quadrant pain radiating to the right shoulder and scapula

44 The physician schedules Mr. S. for an endoscopic retrograde cholangiopancreatography (ERCP). The patient asks the nurse to explain what this is. Which response should the nurse make?

A. "ERCP is an X-ray procedure of the stomach using a contrast medium"
B. "ERCP is an examination of the esophagus, stomach, small intestines, pancreas, and gallbladder through a scope inserted in your mouth"
C. "ERCP is a noninvasive procedure using high-frequency sound waves, which are aimed into the body and recorded as they reflect back"
D. "ERCP is an X-ray procedure of the pancreas and gallbladder using a contrast medium"

45 Mr. S. experiences steatorrhea, which refers to:

A. Bulky, greasy, foul-smelling stools
B. Hard, formed, clay-colored stools
C. Black or tarry stools
D. Formed, streaked, mucoid stools

46 While bathing Mr. S., the nurse notices muscle twitching and irritability of the nervous system. This is probably caused by a decrease in:

A. Potassium
B. Ammonia
C. Calcium
D. Sodium

47 The physician orders meperidine (Demerol) for Mr. S.'s abdominal discomfort. This is the drug of choice because it:

A. Does not cause nausea and vomiting
B. Causes less spasm of the smooth muscles of the pancreatic ducts
C. Does not cause sedation of the central nervous system
D. Does not cause sedation of the peripheral nerve endings

SITUATION

Mrs. A., a 32-year-old mother of two, is admitted with ulcerative colitis. She has been hospitalized many times with the same problem; medical management has been unsuccessful. She is anorectic and anemic and has lost 20 lb. She tells the nurse that she has constant abdominal pain and bloody diarrhea. The nurse prepares Mrs. A. for an ileos-

tomy. The physician orders large doses of kanamycin (Kantrex) P.O. for several days.

Questions 48 to 52 refer to this situation.

48 Mrs. A. asks the nurse what the medication will do. The nurse's best response would be that kanamycin:

A. Helps prevent infection resulting from surgery
B. Is routinely given to all surgical patients before surgery
C. Cleans the bowel of bacteria because it is poorly absorbed from the intestine
D. Causes diarrhea and cleans the intestine before surgery

49 After Mrs. A.'s ileostomy surgery, the nurse assesses her abdomen and notices that the stoma is purplish red. The nurse should:

A. Reassure the patient that this is the normal color
B. Watch the stoma for any further changes in color
C. Apply warm soaks to the stoma to improve circulation
D. Report this finding to the physician immediately

50 Mrs. A. has a large amount of drainage from her stoma. Blood tests reveal a serum sodium level of 135 mEq/liter, a serum potassium level of 2.5 mEq/liter, and a serum chloride level of 98 mEq/liter. Which food combination would be most beneficial?

A. Liver, oysters, and green, leafy vegetables
B. Bananas, orange juice, and cereals
C. Celery, carrots, and fish
D. Clams, oysters, and sardines

51 Which topic would *not* be discussed during the nurse's patient-teaching session with Mrs. A.?

A. Application of the stomal appliance
B. The procedure for daily irrigations
C. Foods to eat and avoid
D. Information on self-help groups

52 Mrs. A.'s roommate has a colostomy. Mrs. A. asks the nurse to explain the difference between an ileostomy and a colostomy. The nurse's best response would be:

A. "An ileostomy is temporary; a colostomy is permanent"
B. "An ileostomy is always done for cancer; a colostomy is only done for ulcerative colitis"
C. "Ileostomy stool is liquid and not controllable; colostomy stool is formed and more controllable"
D. "Ileostomy stool is not irritating to the skin; colostomy stool is very irritating to the skin"

SITUATION

S., a 19-year-old woman with newly diagnosed Type I diabetes mellitus, is being discharged today.

Questions 53 to 55 refer to this situation.

53 Which statement indicates a need for further instruction?

A. "I will test my blood glucose before each meal and before bedtime"
B. "I don't like injecting insulin in my arms and legs; I will just use my abdomen"
C. "I will remember to eat after taking my insulin"
D. "It is important for me to follow a specific diet for the rest of my life"

54 During afternoon rounds, the nurse notes that S. appears to be alert but weak, nervous, and diaphoretic. Her lunch tray is untouched. When the nurse questions S. about this, she states she has just returned from a long physical therapy session. The nurse should:

A. Explain how exercise increases glucose uptake
B. Administer insulin immediately
C. Start a normal saline solution I.V. line immediately
D. Warn her against "sneaking" candy during physical therapy

55 Which topic would *not* be discussed during the nurse's patient-teaching session with S.?

A. Insulin injection techniques and signs and symptoms of hyperglycemia and hypoglycemia
B. The need to take oral hypoglycemic medications at the same time each day
C. The diet and exercise plan
D. Long-term complications of diabetes

SITUATION

Mr. H., a 54-year-old patient who has been transferred from telemetry monitoring to direct monitoring in the medical unit, complains of chest pain. The physician has ruled out myocardial infarction (MI) and diagnoses stable angina pectoris.

Questions 56 to 60 refer to this situation.

56 When describing his pain to the nurse, Mr. H. would most likely say that it:

A. Is located over his left nipple
B. Feels like a stab in the chest
C. Awakens him out of sound sleep
D. Feels like his chest and throat are being squeezed

57 During rounds, the nurse finds Mr. H. sitting on the edge of his bed, clutching his chest. He tells the nurse he is having a heart attack. The nurse's first action should be to:

A. Administer the nitroglycerin (Nitro-Bid) kept at the patient's bedside
B. Administer oxygen via nasal cannula at 2 liters/minute
C. Obtain apical pulse and respiratory rates
D. Call for an immediate electocardiogram to document ischemia during the episode

58 Which topic of discussion is *not* essential during the nurse's patient-teaching session with Mr. H.?

A. Diet counseling
B. Common surgical interventions
C. Influence of sexual activity on angina
D. Stress management

59 The physician orders 1" of nitroglycerin ointment every 6 hours for Mr. H. Which nursing action is of primary importance when administering this drug?

A. Applying it to a hairless area of skin
B. Covering it with a piece of plastic wrap after each application
C. Using the same administration technique with each application
D. Applying it to the upper back or chest to improve absorption

60 Which rationale for the use of calcium channel blockers to treat angina is *not* correct?

A. They interfere with vasoconstriction and reduce vasospasm
B. They increase cardiac output and myocardial oxygenation through inotropic and chronotropic effects
C. They allow prolonged diastole, which augments coronary artery perfusion
D. They help balance myocardial oxygen supply and demand

SITUATION

Mrs. S., a 56-year-old patient on the surgical unit, had a total abdominal hysterectomy 2 days ago. She has a history of angina and non-insulin-dependent diabetes mellitus. She has been walking, tolerates a soft diet, and has audible bowel sounds. Her vital signs have been stable, revealing a temperature of 98.9° F (37.2° C), a pulse rate of 78 beats/minute, a respiratory rate of 15 breaths/minute, and a blood pressure of 134/86 mm Hg.

Questions 61 to 66 refer to this situation.

---

61 Mrs. S. suddenly calls the nurse into her room, complaining of severe indigestion. She is pale, diaphoretic, and says she knows "something dreadful is going to happen." Her pulse is 120 beats/minute and thready; her respiratory rate, 22 breaths/minute; and her blood pressure, 100/60 mm Hg. The nurse's first action should be to:

A. Administer 6 oz of orange juice and call the physician immediately
B. Administer an antacid and call the physician immediately
C. Call the physician immediately
D. Call the physician and ask him to prescribe a stronger analgesic

62 Mrs. S. is transferred to the cardiac care unit with a diagnosis of inferior wall MI. Within the first 24 hours, cardiac enzyme tests should show:

A. Normal serum lactate dehydrogenase (LDH) levels, elevated serum creatine phosphokinase (CPK) levels, and elevated serum aspartate aminotransferase (AST; formerly serum glutamic-oxaloacetic transaminase) levels
B. Slightly elevated serum LDH levels, elevated serum CPK levels, and elevated serum AST levels
C. Normal serum LDH levels, normal serum CPK levels, and elevated serum AST levels
D. Slightly elevated serum LDH levels, elevated serum CPK levels, and normal serum AST levels

63 Because of the nature of Mrs. S.'s MI, the nurse should assess for:

A. Cardiogenic shock
B. Pulmonary embolism
C. Arrhythmias
D. Congestive heart failure

64 Which treatment goal should be the nurse's chief concern during the acute phase of Mrs. S.'s illness?

A. Relieving anxiety
B. Decreasing tissue perfusion
C. Decreasing cardiac output
D. Relieving pain

65 Four days after her admission, Mrs. S. is discharged from the cardiac care unit to her original unit. She is quiet, answers questions in monosyllables, and is reluctant to perform any activity without nursing assistance. Which statement by the nurse would best help determine the reason for the patient's behavior?

A. "Why aren't you your usual cheerful self, Mrs. S.?"
B. "You seem very quiet, Mrs. S."
C. "Are you depressed, Mrs. S.?"
D. "In a few days you'll start feeling like your old self; most patients feel depressed after they've had a heart attack"

66 The physician will probably schedule a stress test for Mrs. S. to determine:

A. Her functional capacity, which helps health care personnel plan an appropriate rehabilitation program
B. The risk of further infarctions
C. The extent of necrosis caused by the infarction
D. Her ability to return to her normal activities of daily living after discharge

---

SITUATION

Mrs. J., a 40-year-old homemaker with a recent diagnosis of rheumatoid arthritis, has come to the clinic for a follow-up visit.

Questions 67 to 69 refer to this situation.

67 When describing rheumatoid arthritis to Mrs. J., the nurse should tell her that it is:

A. A short-term health problem involving only the joints
B. More common in men than women
C. An immune-mediated disease involving the connective tissues
D. A chronic, diffuse connective tissue disease affecting multiple organs

68 Periodic nursing assessment of Mrs. J. should include:

A. Inspection, palpation, and nursing history about each of the involved joint areas
B. Listening for cues about her self-image and financial concerns
C. Determining her weight gain or loss since the last visit
D. A systematic review of body systems, coping abilities, and financial concerns

69 Mrs. J. calls the nurse at the clinic early one morning, complaining of dizziness and ringing in her ears. Which question should the nurse ask first?

A. "Have you taken your aspirin this morning?"
B. "Did you just get up?"
C. "How is your appetite?"
D. "Are you upset about something?"

SITUATION

Mr. O., age 62, visits his physician complaining of severe indigestion and lower back pain. His physician palpates an abdominal mass and auscultates an abdominal bruit. Mr. O. is immediately admitted to a surgical unit for evaluation. An aortogram reveals an aneurysm.

Questions 70 to 72 refer to this situation.

70 Which complication represents the greatest threat to Mr. O. before his abdominal aortic aneurysm is surgically repaired?

A. Rupture
B. Embolism in the foot
C. Aortic dissection
D. Cerebrovascular accident

71 When caring for Mr. O. preoperatively, the nurse should assess periodically for:

A. Sudden headache
B. Increased anxiety
C. Increased blood pressure with decreased pulse rate
D. Decreased blood pressure with increased pulse rate

72 When the nurse attempts to teach Mr. O. about his impending surgery, he tells her, "I don't want to know anything until I wake up." The nurse's best response would be:

A. "Are you frightened, Mr. O.?"
B. "You will recover much more quickly if you listen to what we have to say"
C. "It's normal to have anxiety before surgery as serious as this, Mr. O."
D. "If you don't want to hear this right now, Mr. O., it's all right. We are here if you need any questions answered"

SITUATION

Mr. J., age 45, has a history of chronic alcohol abuse. He is admitted to the hospital with liver enlargement, ascites, jaundice, weakness, anorexia, and fluid retention. The physician diagnoses Laënnec's cirrhosis of the liver.

Questions 73 to 77 refer to this situation.

73 When caring for Mr. J., the nurse should know how individual drugs are metabolized by the body before she administers them because:

A. The liver may be unable to excrete the drugs
B. The patient already has a substance abuse problem
C. The kidneys may be unable to excrete the drugs
D. The drugs may alter the patient's level of consciousness

74 Which dietary intervention is *not* likely to be instituted for treating Mr. J.'s anorexia and malnourishment?

A. A fat-free diet
B. Vitamin supplements
C. A moderately high carbohydrate intake
D. A daily intake of 2,000 to 3,000 calories

75 Which complication would *not* result from advanced cirrhosis of the liver?

A. Ascites
B. Asthma
C. GI bleeding
D. Encephalopathy

76 During a patient-teaching session with Mr. J., the nurse cautions him about activities that increase intrathoracic pressure—such as coughing or straining at stool—because they may:

A. Cause jaundice
B. Increase leg swelling
C. Induce rupture of the esophageal varices
D. Lead to encephalopathy

77 The physician inserts a balloon-tamponade (Sengstaken-Blakemore) tube to stop the bleeding from Mr. J.'s esophageal varices. The physician may release the balloon pressure periodically to:

A. Prevent esophageal tissue damage
B. Improve patient comfort
C. Prevent the development of additional bleeding varices
D. Suction saliva from the oropharynx

SITUATION

Ms. W., age 45, has a recent diagnosis of systemic lupus erythematosus. The physician orders 15 mg of prednisone every other day.

Questions 78 and 79 refer to this situation.

---

78 The nurse should instruct Ms. W. to take her prednisone:

A. At bedtime
B. After lunch
C. With food before 8 a.m.
D. 1 hour before any meal

---

79 Ms. W. plans to go to the beach for vacation. Which instruction should the nurse give her?

A. "There are no restrictions on your activities, but plan rest periods"
B. "Get some sun, but limit your exposure time because sunburn can occur quickly"
C. "Remember to pack your medications in your suitcase when you leave"
D. "Wear a sunscreen lotion and avoid exposure to the sunlight"

SITUATION

Mr. B. is receiving 40% oxygen via a Venturi mask. Arterial blood gas (ABG) analysis reveals a pH of 7.18, a partial pressure of carbon dioxide in arterial blood ($PaCO_2$) of 66 mm Hg, a partial pressure of oxygen in arterial blood (PaO_2) of 53 mm Hg, and a bicarbonate (HCO_3^-) level of 24.3 mEq/liter.

Questions 80 and 81 refer to this situation.

---

80 Mr. B.'s ABG levels indicate that he is in:

A. Respiratory alkalosis
B. Respiratory acidosis
C. Compensated respiratory acidosis
D. Metabolic alkalosis

---

81 To treat Mr. B., the nurse should:

A. Administer sodium bicarbonate I.V.
B. Increase the fraction of inspired oxygen to correct hypoxemia
C. Begin incentive spirometry therapy
D. Provide supportive mechanical ventilation

SITUATION

Mrs. T., a 65-year-old patient with breast cancer, is scheduled for a modified radical mastectomy.

Questions 82 and 83 refer to this situation.

---

82 A modified radical mastectomy involves:

A. Removal of breast tissue, lymph nodes, and the small pectoralis muscle
B. Segmental wedge resection of breast tissue and nodal dissection
C. Removal of the breast only
D. Removal of both pectoralis muscles, lymph nodes, and breast tissue

---

83 Because Mrs. T. is postmenopausal and estrogen receptors are positive, the physician plans hormone manipulation after her surgery. Which drug will the physician probably order?

A. Vincristine (Oncovin)
B. Fluorouracil (5-fluorouracil)
C. Tamoxifen (Nolvadex)
D. Methotrexate

SITUATION

Mrs. P., age 76, is admitted to the medical unit with joint pain, mild tenderness, and right knee enlargement. Her admission diagnosis is osteoarthritis.

Questions 84 and 85 refer to this situation.

---

84 Which assessment finding is *not* likely for Mrs. P.'s affected knee?

A. Crepitation on movement
B. Limited range of motion
C. Atrophy of surrounding muscles
D. Painless subcutaneous nodules near the joint

---

85 During morning rounds, the nurse notices that Mrs. P.'s right knee is acutely swollen and painful. Besides administering an appropriate analgesic, the nurse should:

A. Apply moist heat
B. Apply a cold pack
C. Continue isometric and range-of-motion exercises
D. Allow Mrs. P. out of bed with partial weight bearing

SITUATION

Mr. X. is admitted to the hospital with third-degree burns over 10% of his body-surface area. Initial medical treatment includes normal saline solution I.V. and antibiotic therapy; the physician later orders a high-calorie diet, although Mr. X.'s weight exceeds his ideal body weight.

Questions 86 to 88 refer to this situation.

86 Which treatment objective is *not* necessary to prevent or minimize further complications?

A. Preventing and controlling infection
B. Supplying nutritional needs, including replacement fluids and electrolytes
C. Encouraging the patient to attain his ideal body weight
D. Providing psychological support

87 Besides a high-calorie diet, Mr. X. requires:

A. Vitamin D supplements
B. Iron supplements
C. A high protein intake
D. Calcium supplements

88 Which nutritional measure may *not* be appropriate for Mr. X.?

A. Frequent feedings
B. Between-meal feedings
C. Oral feedings only
D. A high intake of complete protein

SITUATION

C., a 20-year-old nursing student, has been hospitalized with ulcerative colitis for the fourth time in a year. During lunch, C. angrily pushes her food tray onto the floor. She exclaims, "I'm sick of this food; it doesn't help me anyway. I can't take any more of this."

Questions 89 and 90 refer to this situation.

89 The nurse's best response to C. would be:

A. "Ulcerative colitis is not easy to live with"
B. "You have a right to be frustrated, but this does not help matters"
C. "You are doing much better than you realize"
D. "It sounds like you're giving up, that you can't take any more"

90 To help C. comply with her diet, the nurse should:

A. Explain the importance of diet in treating ulcerative colitis
B. Convince or force the patient to eat
C. Allow the patient to select foods that she finds appetizing
D. Allow the patient to eat all she can tolerate

SITUATION

Mrs. J., an obese 28-year-old mother of three children, is admitted to the hospital with a diagnosis of acute abdomen. The physician performs an exploratory laparotomy and appendectomy.

Questions 91 to 98 refer to this situation.

91 Mrs. J.'s risk factors for proper wound healing include:

A. Age
B. Obesity
C. Sex
D. Previous pregnancies

92 Mrs. J. is admitted to the recovery room with an oral airway, a nasogastric (NG) tube, two bulb suction (Jackson-Pratt) drains, and lactated Ringer's solution infusing intravenously. The nurse's first action should be to:

A. Check the NG tube for patency and drainage
B. Check blood pressure and pulse rate and compare them to the baseline readings
C. Check the incision site for signs of bleeding
D. Check the airway for patency and assess respirations

93 When Mrs. J. returns to the nursing unit, the physician orders NG tube irrigations. To check the tube for correct placement, the nurse should:

A. Use a syringe to gently aspirate secretions from the tube
B. Inject 10 to 20 ml of irrigating fluid while auscultating the left upper quadrant of the abdomen
C. Check that the tube is securely anchored to the patient's nose
D. Place the end of the tube below the level of the bed and look for back flow

94 Which substance should *not* be recorded as fluid output on the intake and output sheet?

A. Watery stool
B. Mucus suctioned from the oropharynx and nasopharynx
C. Fluid returned after NG tube irrigation
D. Serosanguinous drainage from the Jackson-Pratt drains

95 The physician orders the removal of Mrs. J.'s NG tube and places her on a clear liquid diet. Which foods would be included on this diet?

A. Gelatin, chicken broth, and coffee
B. Beef broth, gelatin, and ginger ale
C. Beef broth, gelatin, and apple juice
D. Chicken broth, gelatin, and tea

96 When helping Mrs. J. out of bed for the first time after surgery, the nurse should *not:*

A. Elevate the head of the bed for 10 minutes beforehand
B. Ask another staff member to assist the nurse if needed
C. Ask the patient's husband to help her out of bed to involve him in her care
D. Check the patient's vital signs before and after she gets up

97 The physican orders deep-breathing and coughing exercises for Mrs. J. Which nursing instruction would help improve cough effectiveness and patient comfort?

A. "When coughing, lie flat in bed with a pillow under the lower back to elevate the lower lungs and assist with drainage"
B. "Sit up in bed, hold a pillow against the abdominal incision, take several deep breaths, and cough forcibly"
C. "When coughing, lie on either side with a pillow under your waist to elevate the lower lungs and assist with drainage"
D. "Sit up in bed with your stomach against the overbed table, take several deep breaths, and cough forcibly"

98 The nurse notes subjective symptoms of wound infection in Mrs. J. These symptoms include:

A. A fever 3 or more days after surgery
B. An elevated white blood cell count
C. Increased swelling and erythema
D. Persistent incisional pain and a feeling of general malaise

The physician removes the staples from Mrs. J.'s incision site and irrigates the wound, then orders wound and skin precautions and application of wet-to-dry dressings.

Questions 99 and 100 continue the situation.

99 When changing Mrs. J.'s dressings, the nurse should:

A. Seal the soiled dressing in a plastic bag, wash her hands, and don sterile gloves before applying the new dressing
B. Take the patient to the treatment room for each dressing change to provide a clean environment
C. Wash her hands, remove the soiled dressing, and touch only the corners of the new dressing while applying it
D. Don a gown, mask, and gloves before removing the soiled dressing

100 Mrs. J.'s wound will heal by:

A. Primary intention
B. Secondary intention
C. Tertiary intention
D. Regeneration

Answer sheet

	A B C D		A B C D		A B C D		A B C D
1	○ ○ ○ ○	31	○ ○ ○ ○	61	○ ○ ○ ○	91	○ ○ ○ ○
2	○ ○ ○ ○	32	○ ○ ○ ○	62	○ ○ ○ ○	92	○ ○ ○ ○
3	○ ○ ○ ○	33	○ ○ ○ ○	63	○ ○ ○ ○	93	○ ○ ○ ○
4	○ ○ ○ ○	34	○ ○ ○ ○	64	○ ○ ○ ○	94	○ ○ ○ ○
5	○ ○ ○ ○	35	○ ○ ○ ○	65	○ ○ ○ ○	95	○ ○ ○ ○
6	○ ○ ○ ○	36	○ ○ ○ ○	66	○ ○ ○ ○	96	○ ○ ○ ○
7	○ ○ ○ ○	37	○ ○ ○ ○	67	○ ○ ○ ○	97	○ ○ ○ ○
8	○ ○ ○ ○	38	○ ○ ○ ○	68	○ ○ ○ ○	98	○ ○ ○ ○
9	○ ○ ○ ○	39	○ ○ ○ ○	69	○ ○ ○ ○	99	○ ○ ○ ○
10	○ ○ ○ ○	40	○ ○ ○ ○	70	○ ○ ○ ○	100	○ ○ ○ ○
11	○ ○ ○ ○	41	○ ○ ○ ○	71	○ ○ ○ ○		
12	○ ○ ○ ○	42	○ ○ ○ ○	72	○ ○ ○ ○		
13	○ ○ ○ ○	43	○ ○ ○ ○	73	○ ○ ○ ○		
14	○ ○ ○ ○	44	○ ○ ○ ○	74	○ ○ ○ ○		
15	○ ○ ○ ○	45	○ ○ ○ ○	75	○ ○ ○ ○		
16	○ ○ ○ ○	46	○ ○ ○ ○	76	○ ○ ○ ○		
17	○ ○ ○ ○	47	○ ○ ○ ○	77	○ ○ ○ ○		
18	○ ○ ○ ○	48	○ ○ ○ ○	78	○ ○ ○ ○		
19	○ ○ ○ ○	49	○ ○ ○ ○	79	○ ○ ○ ○		
20	○ ○ ○ ○	50	○ ○ ○ ○	80	○ ○ ○ ○		
21	○ ○ ○ ○	51	○ ○ ○ ○	81	○ ○ ○ ○		
22	○ ○ ○ ○	52	○ ○ ○ ○	82	○ ○ ○ ○		
23	○ ○ ○ ○	53	○ ○ ○ ○	83	○ ○ ○ ○		
24	○ ○ ○ ○	54	○ ○ ○ ○	84	○ ○ ○ ○		
25	○ ○ ○ ○	55	○ ○ ○ ○	85	○ ○ ○ ○		
26	○ ○ ○ ○	56	○ ○ ○ ○	86	○ ○ ○ ○		
27	○ ○ ○ ○	57	○ ○ ○ ○	87	○ ○ ○ ○		
28	○ ○ ○ ○	58	○ ○ ○ ○	88	○ ○ ○ ○		
29	○ ○ ○ ○	59	○ ○ ○ ○	89	○ ○ ○ ○		
30	○ ○ ○ ○	60	○ ○ ○ ○	90	○ ○ ○ ○		

Answers and rationales

1 Correct answer—**D**

Recent studies indicate that shaving the incision site in the operating room lowers the infection rate. Some authorities recommend against using prophylactic antibiotics after surgery; it increases resistance to the drug and decreases the effectiveness of the antibiotic if the patient becomes ill later. The patient can wash his hair the night before or the morning of surgery; this will not affect the risk of postoperative infection unless the cranium is the operative site. The nurse should encourage the patient to shower before surgery for hygienic reasons; however, this action is not as effective in preventing postoperative infection as shaving the incision site because it does not remove hair, which harbors bacteria, from the body.

2 Correct answer—**B**

Allowing the patient nothing to eat or drink for 8 hours before surgery helps prevent vomiting and aspiration of food during anesthesia induction, which may be life-threatening or lead to pneumonia; reduces the possibility of bowel obstruction; and prevents contamination of the surgical area from fecal material during intestinal surgery. Prohibiting the patient from eating and drinking does not promote nutritional status or promote blood supply to the surgical site. Paralytic ileus may result from fluid and electrolyte imbalance, effects of general anesthesia, or immobility; it is not related to food and fluid intake before surgery.

3 Correct answer—**C**

Release of antidiuretic hormone by the posterior pituitary during the stress response causes water retention for 48 to 72 hours postoperatively. Growth hormone, prolactin, and insulin regulate glucose and insulin balance rather than directly affecting fluid retention or diuresis. The release of growth hormone and prolactin during the stress response causes decreased insulin release; the blood glucose level then increases to meet energy needs. The adrenal medulla's secretion of epinephrine causes mobilization of glycogen stores in the liver. The adrenal cortex's secretion of glucocorticoids stimulates gluconeogenesis by the liver.

4 Correct answer—**D**

Approximately 50% of patients presenting with hyperosmolar nonketotic syndrome (HNKS) are elderly, undiagnosed diabetics. Elderly patients tend to tolerate polydipsia and polyuria longer, dismissing these symptoms as signs of aging. Severe dehydration follows with little or no ketosis. The hyperosmolar state causes cells to shrink, resulting in mental status changes. Blood glucose levels in HNKS are extremely elevated—over 800 mg/dl. Insulin shock, or hypoglycemia, refers to a blood glucose level under 60 mg/dl. With diabetic ketoacidosis (DKA), plasma ketones would be present. DKA most often occurs in patients with undiagnosed Type I diabetes or those who omit their daily insulin injections. An acute lack of insulin causes glucose accumulation in the blood. Breakdown of fat leads to increased concentrations of free fatty acids, which are converted by the liver to ketones.

5 Correct answer—B

This patient is experiencing DKA; insulin and fluids are essential in the treatment of DKA. Low-dose insulin infusion is effective and associated with less hypoglycemia and hypokalemia than that associated with high-dose insulin infusion. Administering dextrose 5% in water would further increase blood glucose levels. Increased oral fluid intake cannot correct the severe dehydration of DKA. Regular insulin, which takes effect in 2 to 4 hours, is required to lower blood glucose levels and reduce ketosis; isophane insulin suspension (NPH), which takes effect in 8 or more hours, is too slow-acting to be useful. Aerobic exercise is unsafe when blood glucose levels exceed 250 mg/dl; muscles do not get the fuel they need during exercise (glucose), and the exercise further raises the blood glucose level by converting glycogen to glucose.

6 Correct answer—D

The best way to evaluate long-term diabetes control is to monitor the glycosylated hemoglobin (hemoglobin A_{1C}) level. Glycosylated hemoglobin results from the permanent attachment of glucose molecules to hemoglobin A; the amount of glycosylation directly correlates with blood glucose levels. This test reflects the average blood glucose level for the preceding 1 to 3 months before the test. Home blood glucose levels, urine tests, and the fasting blood glucose test only monitor the blood glucose level at the time of collection; they cannot be used to evaluate long-term therapy.

7 Correct answer—B

Visceral neuropathy leads to sexual impotence in about half of all diabetic men over age 50; impotence may develop from a combination of autonomic neuropathy affecting the parasympathetic sacral nerve fibers and decreased blood flow to the penis from microvascular changes. Diabetic men typically have adequate endocrine function, and their testosterone levels are normal. Better control of the blood glucose level may help correct impotency. Confining sexual activity to the morning is appropriate for a patient with cardiac problems, not impotency caused by diabetes.

8 Correct answer—B

If a diabetic patient is unconscious and the cause may be hypoglycemia or hyperglycemia, the nurse should always administer dextrose 50% to raise the glucose level; the brain can tolerate an extremely high blood glucose level longer than a low level. Insulin lowers the blood glucose level; if unconsciousness resulted from hypoglycemia, insulin would further aggravate the condition. The patient would require cardiopulmonary resuscitation only if he were not breathing and did not have a pulse; the question did not say this was the case. The nurse should not administer normal saline solution before determining hyperglycemia to be the cause of unconsciousness.

9 Correct answer—D

Cardiac output is the amount of blood ejected from the left ventricle into the aorta per minute; it equals the stroke volume times the heart rate. The amount of tension the ventricle must develop during contraction to eject blood from the left ventricle into the aorta is called the afterload. The amount of blood ejected by the left ventricle into the aorta per beat is the stroke volume. The amount of blood ejected by the left ventricle necessary to adequately perfuse the body is not a measurable quantity; the requirement changes constantly with the body's demand and supply.

10 Correct answer—C

The PR interval represents the period of impulse conduction between the sinoatrial node and the ventricular musculature. The period of ventricular depolarization is represented by the QRS complex on an electrocardiogram (ECG). The period of atrial depolarization is represented by the P wave. Impulse conduction between the atrioventricular node and the ventricular septum is so rapid that a basic ECG cannot detect it.

11 Correct answer—A

The R-on-T phenomenon, which appears near the peak or deflection of T waves, frequently precipitates ventricular tachycardia. The R-on-T phenomenon is a type of premature ventricular contraction. These arrhythmias occur during the relative refractory (vulnerable) period of the depolarization-repolarization cycle; they occur without a P wave and earlier than the next organized complex should occur. Premature atrial contractions and junctional rhythm cause changes in the P wave. Idioventricular rhythm causes changes in the QRS complex.

12 Correct answer—A

Bilateral left hemianopia causes vision loss in the left visual field of both eyes; the patient must learn to compensate for this by scanning (turning his head to the left and back to view all his surroundings with the right visual fields). If the hemianopia resulted from a cerebrovascular accident, the right side of the patient's body would probably be impaired, making rehabilitation techniques useful; however, they would not help the patient's visual problem even if this information applied. Because the right side of the visual field is intact in both eyes, the patient should not wear frosted glasses over his left eye; this would eliminate that field of vision. Hemianopia results from optic nerve damage, not from injury to eye muscles; ocular exercises would not improve this type of injury.

13 Correct answer—B

The inability to communicate by speech or writing or to understand spoken or written language is called aphasia. Apraxia is the inability to initiate movement on command. Dysarthria is the inability to move the muscles of the mouth and throat. Agnosia is the inability to name objects.

14 Correct answer—B

A weight reduction would indicate removal of excess fluid and wastes. The volume of the outflow dialysate should be greater than that of the inflow dialysate. The quality of respirations would not accurately indicate therapeutic effectiveness of peritoneal dialysis, although moist respirations may indicate fluid retention. Redness near the catheter site indicates inflammation and possible infection; it does not indicate whether peritoneal dialysis has achieved its desired effect.

15 Correct answer—A

Cloudiness of the drained dialysate is the earliest sign of peritonitis. A slow output rate indicates that the catheter is positioned incorrectly or obstructed by fibrin. Redness of the skin near the catheter indicates inflammation caused by a foreign body, such as a catheter. Difficulty breathing may indicate respiratory congestion related to pulmonary infection or congestive heart failure, not peritonitis.

16 Correct answer—B

The nurse should avoid using the patient's left arm for I.V. injections to reduce the risk of injuring the graft through accidental puncture or phlebitis. The nurse should take blood pressure readings in the right arm. The patient should avoid lying on his left side; this may cause increased pressure on the graft site. Exercising the arm is appropriate; it promotes circulation through the graft.

17 Correct answer—A

Measuring blood pressure and weight before and after dialysis helps the nurse determine the amount of fluid removed and the effects of dialysis. Daily hemoglobin and hematocrit tests would not provide data about the effects of dialysis. Thirst and dry mouth—common complaints in a patient with end-stage renal disease—do not indicate the effectiveness of dialysis. Inspection of the patient's extremities would not provide accurate data for assessing fluid balance; weight is a more objective measurement.

18 Correct answer—B

The nurse's first action should be to maintain the patient's airway; an inadequate airway may lead to cerebral anoxia and death. The nurse should pad the bed's side rails before any seizure activity to prevent the patient from injuring himself; however, it is not a priority once a seizure has begun. Assessing the patient's level of consciousness and providing privacy for the patient are important nursing actions, but maintaining a patent airway has priority.

19 Correct answer—A

Health care providers should be alert for speech alterations if the lobectomy was performed in the dominant hemisphere; this is typically a temporary complication. Expressive aphasia may be present. Assessment of motor function, temperature regulation, and cognitive function is necessary for all postoperative patients, not just lobectomy patients.

20 Correct answer—B

Hypoproteinemia is associated with an increased risk of wound infection; because protein is essential for synthesis of new tissue, inadequate protein causes more skin breakdown and infection. A positive nitrogen balance, proper nutrition, and optimum weight decrease the risk of postoperative complications; however, weight is not directly related to wound healing.

21 Correct answer—A

Research has shown evidence of decreased postoperative neutrophil levels; neutrophils are primarily responsible for phagocytosis and the destruction of bacteria and other infectious organisms. Malnourishment can aggravate the neutropenia. Faulty sterile technique may lead to postoperative infection regardless of nutritional status. Adequate dietary intake does not always prevent infection. Granulocyte (granular leukocyte) activation is decreased, not increased, after surgery.

22 Correct answer—B

The patient's tachycardia, clammy skin, paleness, and low blood pressure indicate impending hypovolemic shock. Atelectasis would cause an elevated temperature as well as diminished breath sounds, on auscultation, in the affected lung areas. The residual effects of anesthesia may lower the patient's blood pressure but not as low as 80/50 mm Hg; it would probably lower her pulse rate, not raise it. Wound infection is unlikely this soon postoperatively; wound infections more commonly occur on the third postoperative day or later. The low temperature also indicates that this is not a wound infection.

23 Correct answer—D

Soft foods are easier to chew and swallow; because the myasthenia gravis patient's mastication muscles are stronger in the morning, the nurse should serve the main meal of the day at that time. The nurse should not restrict fluids but increase the patient's intake to 3,000 ml or more daily; placing the patient at a 90-degree, not 45-degree, angle facilitates swallowing. Anticholinesterase drugs, if ordered by the physician, should be administered 1 hour before meals to improve muscle strength; liquids and foods should be served hot or cold to trigger the swallowing reflex, improving the patient's ability to swallow. The patient should avoid milk because it stimulates the formation of secretions (also an adverse effect of anticholinesterase drugs), which may compound existing swallowing and airway problems; because weak facial muscles make drinking through a straw difficult or impossible, the nurse should offer fluids to the patient from a cup.

24 Correct answer—A

Easy bruising may indicate a hematopoietic complication; this serious adverse drug effect requires the physician's immediate attention. Decreased facial pain is the expected therapeutic effect of drug therapy for the patient with trigeminal neuralgia; it does not need to be reported immediately to the physician. Dry mouth, a minor adverse effect of phenytoin (Dilantin) therapy, does not require intervention by the physician. Improved sleeping, which indicates that pain has been reduced, is a therapeutic effect the nurse need not report immediately.

25 Correct answer—D

The nurse should assess and document the characteristics of the trigeminal neuralgia pain episode, including precipitating factors, trigger zone locations, description of the pain, and ways the patient tries to prevent episodes (such as keeping away from others and avoiding drafts, oral hygiene, chewing, and shaving). The patient should avoid prolonged use of narcotic medications because of the increased risk of addiction. Jarring movements, such as those in aerobic exercise, may precipitate a pain attack in the patient with trigeminal neuralgia. The patient may prefer frequent, small meals of semiliquid foods served at room temperature; hot or cold foods and fluids may trigger or increase pain.

26 Correct answer—C

To protect all the members of the health team, the nurse should wear gloves and carefully dispose of needles; acquired immunodeficiency syndrome (AIDS) can be transmitted through blood and blood products. Completing laboratory requisitions is a routine nursing function, not a precaution. Careful antiseptic cleaning of the hands and aspirating blood without introducing air into the bloodstream are routine precautions when withdrawing blood from any patient; they are not special precautions with this patient.

27 Correct answer—A

The most critical topic to discuss with the AIDS patient is transmission methods of the virus; because this disease has no cure, it is vital for the patient to understand how to prevent transmitting it to others. The other choices, although important, are not as critical.

28 Correct answer—A

Death from AIDS occurs because of overwhelming opportunistic infection. The human immunodeficiency virus alters immune function; T-cell activity is suppressed, increasing the risk of secondary infection, such as *Pneumocystis carinii* pneumonia or Kaposi's sarcoma. T-cell activity is decreased, not increased. Anaphylaxis and malabsorption are not commonly associated with AIDS.

29 Correct answer—B

The nurse should never administer levodopa with monoamine oxidase inhibitors; combining these drugs can cause a hypertensive crisis. Carbidopa is often given with levodopa to inhibit peripheral conversion of levodopa to dopamine, permitting more levodopa to enter the central nervous system; this allows a lower dosage of levodopa, sharply reducing adverse effects. Anticholinergic drugs, which have an antispasmodic effect, may be given with levodopa; trihexyphenidyl (Artane) is one of these anticholinergic drugs.

30 Correct answer—D

Pulmonary edema refers to the accumulation of fluid in the alveoli of the lungs, resulting from increased hydrostatic pressure forcing fluid across the alveolocapillary membrane; it causes increased pulmonary pressure, not increased intracranial pressure (ICP). Space-occupying masses, such as hematomas, abscesses, and tumors, can cause intracranial hypertension, which can lead to increased ICP. Cerebral edema (an abnormal accumulation of fluid in the intracellular or extracellular space associated with increased brain tissue volume) and hydrocephalus (progressive dilation of the cerebral ventricular system caused by excessive cerebrospinal fluid production and inadequate absorption) may cause increased ICP.

31 Correct answer—A

A respiratory rate of 24 breaths/minute is not life-threatening and does not call for endotracheal intubation and mechanical ventilation. The other choices are guidelines used to determine the need for intubation and ventilatory support. All three findings need not be present before therapy begins, and all clinical and laboratory data should be considered before intubation and ventilation are begun.

32 Correct answer—C

The partial pressure of carbon dioxide in arterial blood ($Paco_2$) should be reduced slowly to an acceptable level (50 to 55 mm Hg). The patient in chronic ventilatory failure (compensated respiratory acidosis) has excess HCO_3^- because of retention by the kidneys. The kidneys take several hours to excrete the excess; if the $Paco_2$ is corrected rapidly, the retained HCO_3^- can cause severe metabolic alkalosis. Administering sodium bicarbonate to a patient with a high HCO_3^- level would worsen metabolic acidosis.

33 Correct answer—C

Because the patient is hypoventilating, acidotic, and unable to take deep breaths and cough, the nurse should prepare for endotracheal tubing and mechanical ventilation to promote respiratory function. Decreasing the fraction of inspired oxygen would lower the partial pressure of oxygen in arterial blood (PaO_2) and worsen hypoxia. Intermittent positive-pressure breathing treatments, chest physiotherapy, and postural drainage would not help correct the immediate problem of hypoventilation.

34 Correct answer—A

The low HCO_3^- level, low pH, and normal $PaCO_2$ indicate metabolic acidosis, commonly seen with diabetic ketoacidosis, severe hypoxemia, lactic acidosis, aspirin overdose, and uremia. Compensated metabolic acidosis would be indicated by a low HCO_3^- level, a normal pH, and a low $PaCO_2$. Respiratory acidosis would be indicated by a normal HCO_3^- level, a low pH, and a high $PaCO_2$. Metabolic alkalosis would be indicated by a high HCO_3^- level, a high pH, and a normal $PaCO_2$.

35 Correct answer—A

The nurse should assess the patient immediately after thyroid surgery for aphonia, the inability to produce vocal sounds. Usually caused by accidental surgical injury to the laryngeal nerve, aphonia is permanent and may lead to serious airway obstruction. A hematoma might cause hoarseness or other changes in the quality of the voice, but this is usually temporary and non-life-threatening; elevated blood pressure typically occurs because of pain, but this is also temporary. Hyperthermia is a more likely complication than hypothermia after thyroid surgery; it is common in thyroid storms. Pneumonia is not a concern immediately after surgery because this postoperative complication does not develop for some time.

36 Correct answer—D

Early indications of hypocalcemia include muscle tremors, numbness and tingling of the extremities and perioral area, and muscle cramps as well as a positive Chvostek's sign (twitching of the upper lip elicited by tapping the cheek) and positive Trousseau's sign (carpopedal spasms from the inflation of a blood pressure cuff around the upper arm). Later signs include tetany, which can progress to generalized tonic-clonic seizures, and laryngeal stridor, which increases the risk of respiratory arrest. Changes in level of consciousness and nausea and vomiting are not indications of hypocalcemia.

37 Correct answer—A

Complaints of cold, pale, painful hands, particularly in the summer, are common in patients with Raynaud's syndrome—paroxysmal vasospasm of the digits. Causing diminished blood flow to the fingers and sometimes the toes, this syndrome is a disorder of the small cutaneous arteries and does not result from venous insufficiency. The angiopathy associated with chronic diabetes is caused by vascular occlusion with arteriosclerosis, not vasospasm; although the effects are similar, angiopathy in a diabetic patient would cause constant, not intermittent, symptoms. Both the veins and arteries are involved. Venous insufficiency is characterized by edema, induration, and discoloration; pain may or may not be present.

38 Correct answer—B

The low pH indicates acidosis; the high $PaCO_2$ indicates the problem is respiratory in nature. Chronic obstructive pulmonary disease (COPD) causes inadequate ventilation, which increases the carbon dioxide level and leads to respiratory acidosis. Respiratory alkalosis would be indicated by a high pH and a low $PaCO_2$. Metabolic alkalosis would be indicated by a high pH and a high HCO_3^- level. Metabolic acidosis would be indicated by a low pH and a low HCO_3^- level.

39 Correct answer—D

Anemia and pulmonary hypotension are not clinical manifestations of COPD. However, dyspnea, intermittent cough, and fatigue after exertion are commonly seen; thick bronchial secretions result from allergies or infectious diseases. Thoracic excursion is reduced by chronic bronchial obstruction, trapped air, and thoracic overdistention, leading to an increased anteroposterior chest diameter (barrel chest). Gradual destruction of the lung parenchyma and loss of the lung's elastic recoil lowers and flattens the diaphragm. Finally, hypoxia causes polycythemia (increased number of red blood cells) rather than anemia; hypoxia and acidosis cause constriction of the pulmonary vessels, resulting in pulmonary hypertension.

40 Correct answer—D

The nurse should report carbon dioxide narcosis immediately to the physician. When pulmonary disease prevents efficient removal of carbon dioxide, the medulla may no longer respond to increased carbon dioxide levels to trigger respiration; instead, decreased oxygen levels may become the most important mechanism in stimulating respirations. Oxygen therapy at 2 to 3 liters/minute may increase the patient's oxygen levels until respirations are no longer triggered, leading to carbon dioxide narcosis. The nurse need not report negative Homans' or Babinski's signs, which are normal assessment findings, or eupnea (normal respirations).

41 Correct answer—C

Depressants commonly cause acute respiratory failure in the patient with COPD; they should not be administered. Bronchodilators relax smooth muscles and assist in opening collapsed air passages. Corticosteroids suppress both the normal and inflammatory response to tissue injury and the protective immune response to invasion by infectious agents. Aerosol agents act as humidifiers, loosening the secretions and helping with expectoration.

42 Correct answer—B

Pursed-lip expiratory breathing prolongs exhalation and helps prevent bronchiolar collapse and trapped air; this technique, coupled with diaphragmatic breathing, gives the patient more control over breathing. Fluid intake should be high, not restricted, to prevent dehydration and drying of secretions. Adequate rest is important, but the patient would probably be more comfortable in the orthopneic position, which relieves dyspnea and aids chest excursion. Performing all his activities at one time will exhaust the patient; activities should be spaced to help conserve the patient's energy so that he can finish them all.

43 Correct answer—A

Abdominal pain is the predominant symptom of chronic and acute pancreatitis; it is usually located in the left upper quadrant and commonly radiates to the back because of the retroperitoneal location of the pancreas. This pain is not relieved with food or antacids. Right lower quadrant pain with rebound tenderness is characteristic of appendicitis. Severe abdominal distention and pain with associated bloody diarrhea typically indicate ulcerative colitis, not pancreatitis. Indigestion and right upper quadrant pain radiating to the right shoulder and scapula indicate cholecystitis.

44 Correct answer—B

The nurse should reply that endoscopic retrograde cholangio-pancreatography is an examination of the esophagus, stomach, small intestines, pancreas, and gallbladder through a scope inserted into the patient's mouth; contrast medium is injected into the common bile duct and pancreatic duct, allowing direct visualization of these structures. An upper GI series is an X-ray examination of the stomach with fluoroscopy using contrast medium. Ultrasound is a noninvasive procedure using high-frequency sound waves. An X-ray procedure of the biliary duct system using a contrast medium is an I.V. cholangiogram.

45 Correct answer—A

Steatorrhea refers to bulky, greasy, foul-smelling, foaming, and yellow-gray stools, which are a common finding in the patient with a malabsorption syndrome. Hard, formed, and clay-colored or light gray stools are a more characteristic finding in patients with biliary obstruction; the stools' color is caused by the absence of urobilin. Black or tarry stools are caused by blood in the upper GI tract; blood entering the lower portion or passing rapidly through the GI tract causes bright or dark red stools. Mucus or pus may appear in the stools of patients with chronic ulcerative colitis.

46 Correct answer—C

Hypocalcemia, one of the most serious complications of pancreatitis, may result in tetany, which causes jerking, irritability, and muscle twitching. Calcium gluconate is usually given to treat symptomatic hypocalcemia. Observing for electrolyte imbalances is a vital part of nursing care for the pancreatitis patient; decreased potassium, ammonia, or sodium levels would not cause muscle twitching or irritability.

47 Correct answer—B

Meperidine (Demerol) is the drug of choice because it causes less spasm of the smooth muscles of the pancreatic ducts than opiate drugs. Meperidine may cause nausea and vomiting and has a sedative effect on central and peripheral nervous system tissue.

48 Correct answer—C

Because kanamycin (Kantrex) is poorly absorbed from the intestine and rarely produces systemic toxicity, it sterilizes the intestine before intestinal surgery. Neomycin (Mycifradin) may be used as well. Preoperative antibiotics are not routinely given to prevent postoperative infection. Kanamycin may cause diarrhea, but diarrhea does not clean the intestine.

49 Correct answer—D

A stoma that is dark red to purple, rather than the normal medium red color, indicates inadequate blood supply to the stoma or bowel and should be reported immediately to the physician; the nurse should not wait to see if further changes develop. Applying warm soaks would cause vasodilation of the external portion of the stoma but would not improve the inadequate blood supply to the bowel or the internal portion of the stoma.

50 Correct answer—B

Because the laboratory results indicate hypokalemia, the patient should eat foods high in potassium, such as bananas, orange juice, and cereals. Liver, oysters, and green, leafy vegetables are good sources of iron. Celery, carrots, and fish are high in sodium. Clams, oysters, and sardines are high in iodine.

51 Correct answer—B

Because ileostomies are not irrigated, patient teaching would not cover any procedure for daily irrigation. The ileostomy patient must be taught how to apply and manage the appliance before discharge. The patient needs information on self-care techniques and emotional support to adjust to her new method of toileting; information about possible complications, dietary considerations, need for medical monitoring, and the availability of support or self-help group services in the community provide for these needs.

52 Correct answer—C

The consistency of stool is different for an ileostomy and a colostomy because of the location of the stoma; ileostomy stool is liquid or semiliquid, contains digestive enzymes that may be extremely irritating to the skin, and is uncontrollable. The individual must wear a collection bag over the stoma. Colostomy stool is semiformed or formed; the patient may not need a collection pouch. A colostomy may be temporary or permanent and is usually performed for perforating diverticulitis, trauma, or cancers. An ileostomy is permanent; it may be performed for ulcerative colitis or Crohn's disease.

53 Correct answer—B

The patient's statement about using only the abdomen for insulin injection indicates a need for further instruction; insulin injections should be rotated daily to prevent atrophy or hypertrophy of the skin. Repeated injections in the same site may lead to slow and erratic absorption of insulin from a hypertrophied area. Testing the blood glucose before each meal and before bedtime is appropriate in home blood glucose monitoring for those with Type I diabetes mellitus. Hypoglycemic reactions commonly result from the patient not eating after insulin administration. Diet is critical in diabetes therapy because it determines how much glucose load the pancreas receives.

54 Correct answer—A

The nurse should explain how exercise increases glucose uptake. Exercise increases the patient's sensitivity to insulin, lowering the blood glucose level. She is experiencing a mild to moderate hypoglycemic reaction, probably caused by extra exercise and missing a meal. Eating foods high in glucose will help relieve her symptoms; 6 oz of orange juice provides the fastest form of carbohydrate to raise the blood glucose level. The patient should eat her lunch now to prevent hypoglycemia later in the afternoon. Administering insulin would further lower her blood glucose level, leading to a severe hypoglycemic reaction. Normal saline solution would not provide the glucose the patient needs. Eating candy may result in hyperglycemia, not hypoglycemia.

55 Correct answer—B

Because the patient with Type I diabetes does not use oral hypoglycemic agents, the nurse would not need to discuss administration techniques for these drugs. However, because the patient needs insulin to survive, the nurse should discuss how to inject insulin and how to recognize if the blood glucose level is high or low. Diet and exercise are critical in controlling diabetes. Information about long-term complications of diabetes may motivate the patient to control it better.

56 Correct answer—D

The pain of stable angina pectoris usually is described as squeezing, burning, pressing, choking, aching, or bursting, similar to heartburn or indigestion. The pain typically radiates; it is not usually described as localized over a specific area of the pericardium. The pain of stable angina is rarely described as sharp or stabbing. Nocturnal pain indicates unstable, not stable, angina.

57 Correct answer—A

All of the actions are appropriate, but the first goal in the treatment of an acute anginal attack is pain relief. Administering nitroglycerin (Nitro-Bid) provides pain relief, diminishing anxiety; this decreases oxygen demand and further reduces pain. The nurse may then determine whether the pain results from angina pectoris or a myocardial infarction (MI); failure to achieve pain relief with nitroglycerin indicates an evolving MI.

58 Correct answer—B

Because the nurse does not know whether the patient will require surgery along with current therapy, common surgical interventions should not be discussed at this time. Angina pectoris occurs when myocardial oxygen demand exceeds myocardial oxygen supply; the most common cause of inadequate myocardial perfusion is atherosclerosis, the occlusion of vessels by fatty plaques. Dietary counseling is therefore essential in preventing additional coronary artery occlusion and more angina attacks. Any life-style factors that increase myocardial oxygen demand, such as sexual intercourse and stress, should be discussed with the patient.

59 Correct answer—C

Different techniques in administering nitroglycerin ointment cause differences in absorption and effectiveness; the nurse should use one technique as determined by hospital policy or nursing judgment. Applying the medication over a hairless area of skin is preferred, but this is not as important as consistent administration. Covering the ointment with plastic wrap helps hold the ointment in place, improving absorption; however, this also is not as important as consistent administration. Applying the medication to the chest and back does not improve absorption.

60 Correct answer—B

Calcium channel blockers inhibit transport of calcium ions across myocardial cell membranes, decreasing inotropic and chronotropic activity and cardiac output. Calcium channel blockers have a vasodilatory effect and have been found to reduce coronary artery vasospasm. The decreased inotropic and chronotropic activity reduces the heart rate, allowing prolonged diastole and augmented coronary artery perfusion. The overall effect of these agents is to balance myocardial oxygen supply and demand.

61 Correct answer—C

The nurse should call the physician immediately because the patient is exhibiting classic signs and symptoms of an MI. Clinical manifestations of an MI include crushing, viselike chest pain, sometimes described by the patient as indigestion or a gallbladder attack; feelings of impending doom or severe anxiety; shortness of breath; cyanosis; decreased blood pressure; increased pulse rate; diaphoresis; possible crackles and rhonchi; and cardiac murmur. Orange juice would be helpful for this diabetic patient if she had manifestations of hypoglycemia, not an MI. An antacid would help relieve indigestion, but the assessment findings indicate the patient is experiencing a more severe disorder. Requesting a stronger analgesic is inappropriate until the cause of the patient's condition is determined.

62 Correct answer—B

With an MI, serum lactate hydrogenase (LDH) level elevation occurs within 12 hours, peaks in 48 hours, and lasts 10 to 14 days; serum creatine phosphokinase (CPK) level elevation occurs within 3 to 6 hours, peaks in 12 to 18 hours, and lasts 3 to 4 days; and serum aspartate aminotransferase (AST; formerly serum glutamic-oxaloacetic transaminase) level elevation occurs within 4 to 6 hours, peaks in 24 to 36 hours, and lasts 4 to 7 days. Therefore, cardiac enzyme tests should reveal slightly elevated serum LDH levels, elevated serum CPK levels, and elevated serum AST levels within 24 hours of the patient's MI.

63 Correct answer—C

Inferior wall MIs are more likely than lateral or anterior wall MIs to cause cardiac arrhythmias because the right coronary artery typically provides oxygen for the inferoposterior wall and the sinoatrial and atrioventricular nodes, which are vital in conduction. The nurse should assess for cardiogenic shock, pulmonary embolism, and congestive heart failure in patients with any type of MI, not just inferior wall MI.

64 Correct answer—D

Relieving pain is the most important nursing goal during the acute phase of an MI. Relieving pain reduces anxiety, thereby decreasing myocardial oxygen demand. A decrease in cardiac output results in decreased tissue perfusion, which leads to hypoxia and decreased myocardial oxygen supply. Because anxiety is mostly caused by pain, relieving anxiety is not the nurse's chief concern.

65 Correct answer—B

"You seem very quiet" is a nonthreatening, factual statement; it is a probing statement used to pursue information about the patient's behavior. The nurse should avoid "why" questions, such as why the patient is not as cheerful as usual, because they imply that the patient should be aware of the underlying motivation of her actions or feelings; such questions are threatening and may make the patient think she is being tested. Asking whether the patient is depressed is a closed-ended question; because the patient can answer only "yes" or "no," the question does not encourage the patient to provide additional information. Stating that most patients are depressed after a heart attack dismisses this patient's current feelings.

66 Correct answer—A

In this situation, the physician will probably order a stress test to determine the patient's functional capacity, which helps in planning rehabilitation. Stress test results do not determine the risk of further infarctions or the extent of myocardial necrosis. The stress test alone will not, at this time, determine the patient's ability to return to normal activities of daily living.

67 Correct answer—D

Rheumatoid arthritis is a chronic, systemic connective tissue disease affecting multiple organs; its etiology is unknown. Rheumatoid arthritis is not a short-term health problem, and statistics indicate that its incidence is 2 to 3 times higher in women than men. The relationship between rheumatoid arthritis and the autoimmune responses of the connective tissues of the entire body are speculative.

68 Correct answer—D

A periodic, systemic review of body systems for the patient with rheumatoid arthritis is recommended because the disease may affect multiple systems; to provide holistic care, the nurse should also assess the patient's ability to cope with the chronicity of the disease and discuss the potential and real economic problems of a long-term disability. The other choices are appropriate but incomplete.

69 Correct answer—A

Dizziness and ringing in the ears are symptoms of aspirin overdose; the nurse should ask the patient if she has taken her morning aspirin dose yet and advise her to limit activity while she is dizzy to prevent further injury. If the symptoms do not resolve before the next dose of aspirin is due, the patient may require changes in her drug therapy. The other questions would not provide information directly related to the patient's complaint.

70 Correct answer—A

Rupture is the most serious complication of aneurysm; it causes massive internal hemorrhage, pain, and death for 50% to 75% of patients. Embolism of the foot is a possible complication, but it is not as serious as rupture. An aortic dissection (dissecting aneurysm) is a type of aneurysm, not a complication; it results from longitudinal splitting of the arterial wall and lining, resulting in hematoma formation. Cerebrovascular accident is not a complication of abdominal aortic aneurysm.

71 Correct answer—D

Clinical manifestations of shock, such as decreased blood pressure with increased pulse rate, indicate rupture of the aneurysm. Sudden headache, increased anxiety, and increased blood pressure with decreased pulse rate are not associated with a ruptured aneurysm.

72 Correct answer—C

Recognizing the patient's anxiety and reassuring him it is normal may encourage him to be more open about his feelings and need for additional information. Asking a specific closed-ended question, such as whether the patient is frightened, may cause him to deny his feelings. Recovery does not depend on this information, and telling the patient that listening will improve recovery may make him feel threatened. Providing the information is important according to the right of informed consent; the patient should hear about the procedure, the potential risks and complications, and possible alternatives to make a fully informed decision. However, the nurse must first relieve the patient's anxiety, which prevents effective learning.

73 Correct answer—A

Drugs that are metabolized solely by the liver are commonly contraindicated in patients with decreased hepatic function; the drugs' effects may be unpredictable or prolonged, and they may cause further damage to the liver. For this reason, agents that are partially excreted through the kidneys are preferred. The patient's substance abuse problem in general—rather than the hepatic damage it has caused—is not related to drug metabolism. Alterations in the patient's level of consciousness may be a drug effect not related to drug metabolism; such alterations are not as significant as the unpredictable effects and hepatic damage that may result with drugs metabolized solely by the liver.

74 Correct answer—A

The patient's fat intake should be moderate, but a fat-free diet usually is unnecessary. Vitamin supplements are given to help correct the effects of malnourishment. Carbohydrate intake, as well as protein intake, should be moderately high depending on the degree of liver damage and the danger of encephalopathy. High carbohydrate and protein intake leads to a high calorie intake—2,000 to 3,000 daily.

75 Correct answer—B

Asthma does not result from cirrhosis of the liver. Fibrotic changes in liver cells obstruct the blood flow, blocking portal circulation; the increased pressure leads to ascites and the formation of esophageal varices. Because the liver can no longer excrete ammonia, encephalopathy may result from toxic ammonia levels.

76 Correct answer—C

Increased intrathoracic pressure can contribute to the rupturing of varices. Increased pressure in the portal circulation causes collateral vessels to develop. These vessels become distended and tend to rupture easily, particularly those located in the esophagus. Hemorrhage from esophageal varices may be fatal. The other choices are not caused by increased intrathoracic pressure. Jaundice is caused by excess bilirubin, which the liver cannot break down and excrete. Leg swelling is caused by impaired venous return resulting from the compression of abdominal blood vessels by ascites. Encephalopathy results from toxic ammonia levels.

77 Correct answer—A

The pressure of the balloon on the esophagus stops hemorrhage, but it may also cause esophageal necrosis; releasing the pressure periodically prevents this tissue damage. Releasing the pressure will not improve patient comfort; the tube remains in place, and the patient cannot feel the pressure changes. The pressure changes may lead to the development of additional bleeding varices instead of preventing them; therefore, this technique is controversial. Saliva can be suctioned from the orpharynx without releasing the pressure.

78 Correct answer—C

Taking a glucocorticoid, such as prednisone, in the early morning (before 8 a.m.) rather than at bedtime helps the patient maintain the normal pattern of cortisol production by the adrenal glands. This production peaks during early morning hours; because cortisol production depends on the the body's cortisol level, taking prednisone in the early morning suppresses the patient's endogenous cortisol production. Taking prednisone with food reduces gastric irritation; taking the drug before or after a meal or snack would be less effective.

79 Correct answer—D

Because exposure to ultraviolet light (sunlight and fluorescent lights) can activate systemic lupus erythematosis, the patient should avoid direct exposure to sunlight and wear sunscreen lotion to filter out reflected rays. Giving the patient no restrictions or telling her she can sunbathe for a limited time may lead to dangerous exposure to ultraviolet light. The patient should not pack her medications in her luggage but carry them in her purse or pockets; if the suitcase with her medications was lost, a skipped dose might lead to adrenal crisis.

80 Correct answer—B

The patient's pH of 7.18 is lower than normal (7.35 to 7.45), indicating acidosis; the partial pressure of carbon dioxide in arterial blood ($PaCO_2$) of 66 mm Hg is higher than normal (35 to 45 mm Hg), indicating a problem of the respiratory system. Respiratory alkalosis would be indicated by a high pH and a low $PaCO_2$. Compensated respiratory acidosis would be indicated by an HCO_3^- level higher than the normal (22 to 26 mEq/liter), a low pH, and an elevated $PaCO_2$. Metabolic alkalosis would be indicated by a high pH, a normal $PaCO_2$, and a high HCO_3^- level.

81 Correct answer—D

The patient in respiratory acidosis requires supportive mechanical ventilation to increase the alveolar ventilation; if the patient's condition warrants, an endotracheal tube will be inserted for mechanical ventilation. The nurse should not administer sodium bicarbonate because it breaks down to carbon dioxide; this drug is used to treat metabolic, not respiratory, acidosis. The partial pressure of oxygen in arterial blood (PaO_2) indicates hypoxemia, but increasing the fraction of inspired oxygen without mechanical ventilation will not correct the patient's hypoventilation. Incentive spirometry therapy is not effective unless the patient has adequate ventilatory effort, which this patient does not.

82 Correct answer—A

A modified radical mastectomy for cancer involves the removal of breast tissue, lymph nodes, and the small pectoralis muscle. Segmental wedge resection is not a mastectomy because the breast is not removed; wedge resections are used commonly in other procedures, such as lung surgery, but rarely in breast surgery. Removal of the breast only is used to treat Paget's disease of the nipples. Removal of both pectoralis muscles, lymph nodes, and breast tissue is a radical mastectomy; because this surgery does not prevent axillary extension or parasternal metastasis, this procedure is seldom used.

83 Correct answer—C

Tamoxifen (Nolvadex) is the drug of choice in hormone manipulation for breast cancer. Because many breast tumors (especially in postmenopausal women) contain estrogen receptors, estrogen causes tumor growth; the physician will probably order tamoxifen because it causes fewer adverse effects than other antiestrogen agents. Vincristine (Oncovin), methotrexate, and fluorouracil (5-fluorouracil) are chemotherapeutic agents with major adverse effects; the physician may order chemotherapy if hormone manipulation is ineffective.

84 Correct answer—D

Painless subcutaneous nodules near joints are a clinical manifestation of rheumatoid arthritis, not osteoarthritis; they are caused by friction and pressure. In osteoarthritis, narrowing of the joint space, osteophyte formation, and sclerosis of subchondral bone cause crepitation on movement, pain and stiffness, and limited range of motion to the affected joint; as the joint becomes progressively restricted in motion, the surrounding muscles atrophy.

85 Correct answer—B

Applying a cold pack is appropriate with acute joint swelling; cold applications cause vasoconstriction, which decreases blood flow and helps decrease swelling. Heat application is contraindicated because it causes vasodilation, increasing blood flow and joint swelling. Acutely inflamed joints should not be exercised until swelling subsides to prevent further stress; therefore, isometric and range-of-motion exercises and partial weight bearing are contraindicated.

86 Correct answer—C

Deliberate attempts to lose weight during the early phase of burn therapy would keep the patient in a state of negative nitrogen balance (catabolism); this would further complicate the patient's condition because he needs to rebuild tissue. Infection control is necessary to help ensure proper healing. Fluid and electrolyte replacement helps prevent weight loss, catabolism, and the effects of fluid and electrolyte imbalances. The nurse should provide psychological support for the patient; burns commonly have a negative effect on the patient's body image.

87 Correct answer—C

Besides a high-calorie diet, the patient requires a high protein intake for tissue replacement and growth. Protein losses in burns are significantly increased because of muscle catabolism under stress and protein loss through the burn wound. For effective tissue repair and replacement, the patient needs high calories from foods other than protein; the protein's energy can then be used for repair and growth rather than body maintenance. At least 2 g of protein/kg of body weight, rather than the normal intake of 0.8 g/kg of body weight, is recommended; the patient may eventually require as much as four times the normal intake. The patient's diet should include adequate vitamin D, iron, and calcium; if assessment reveals any deficiencies, the physician decides if supplements are necessary. Supplementation is most likely with iron; this nutrient is lost because of tissue loss and other effects of burns, and the patient may be unable to consume sufficient iron on his diet.

88 Correct answer—C

Depending on various factors, oral feedings alone may not be practical; for example, the burn patient requires such a high caloric intake that he may be unable to eat enough food. The concentrated formulas used in enteral nutrition (tube feedings) and total parenteral nutrition help ensure adequate nutritional intake. Because the burn patient is encouraged to fulfill his nutritional needs through oral feedings as much as possible to prevent trauma from a feeding tube or central venous catheter, the patient requires frequent feedings, including between-meal feedings. His intake of complete protein (containing the nine essential amino acids in the proportion needed for growth) should be high to speed healing.

89 Correct answer—D

This response is an example of reflection, an important therapeutic communication technique; it restates and summarizes the patient's feelings, encouraging her to continue expressing her feelings. Stating that the disease is not easy to live with confirms the patient's difficulties but does not encourage her to further express her feelings. Confirming the difficulty of living with the illness then chastising the patient for her behavior does not encourage the patient to express her feelings; reassuring the patient that she is doing well has the same drawback.

90 Correct answer—C

Because ulcerative colitis causes many food restrictions, the patient should select foods she finds appetizing. The patient may occasionally select a restricted food, but self-selection usually results in greater compliance with the recommended diet. Explaining the importance of the diet is inappropriate at this time because it would increase the patient's frustration with the diet. The nurse should never force the patient to do something or argue that she should do so because such intervention is nontherapeutic; also, the patient has the right to refuse to eat. Allowing the patient to eat all she can tolerate is inappropriate; this action would not relieve the patient's frustration about what she may eat and could lead to inadequate or excessive intake, which may exacerbate ulcerative colitis.

91 Correct answer—B

Wound separation, infection, and impaired wound healing are more likely in an obese patient because fatty tissue has fewer blood vessels. Very young and very old patients are at increased risk for wound healing problems, but this patient's age is not a risk factor. Women do not have a greater risk of wound healing problems than men. Cesarean delivery, not previous pregnancy, is a risk factor for wound healing.

92 Correct answer—D

Airway obstruction is the most common cause of postoperative respiratory distress; assessing respirations is critical in maintaining adequate gas exchange postanesthesia. The nurse should check the nasogastric (NG) tube for patency, obtain the blood pressure and pulse rate, and assess the incision site *after* assessing the patient's airway and respirations.

93 Correct answer—A

The nurse should use a syringe to gently aspirate secretions from the NG tube; obtaining gastric secretions indicates that the tube is placed correctly in the stomach. The nurse may further verify tube placement by auscultating the epigastric area while injecting air (usually less than 50 cc) into the tube; a gurgling sound indicates that the tube is in the stomach. Injecting 10 to 20 ml of fluid would lead to aspiration if the tube were in the lung. External anchoring of the NG tube does not ensure proper internal placement. Checking back flow from gravity is inconclusive; blockage could prevent back flow even if the tube was placed properly.

94 Correct answer—**B**

Oropharyngeal and nasopharyngeal secretions should not be recorded as fluid output; the amount is usually negligible and difficult to differentiate from the solution used to rinse the catheter. Watery stool should be measured and recorded as fluid output. Fluid used to irrigate the NG tube is recorded as intake and any fluid return is recorded as output. Collection containers for Jackson-Pratt drains should be emptied as needed and the amount measured and recorded as output.

95 Correct answer—**C**

A clear liquid diet consists of fluids that are transparent, easy to digest, nonstimulating, and nonirritating; beef and chicken broth, gelatin, and apple juice are examples of such fluids. Coffee, ginger ale, and tea are irritating fluids that stimulate gastric acid secretion.

96 Correct answer—**C**

The first time a postsurgical patient gets out of bed, several nursing assessments are necessary; a family member is not prepared to assume this responsibility. Elevating the head of the bed for 10 minutes beforehand decreases the effort needed to raise the patient to a sitting position, decreases the stress on the abdominal muscles, and provides time for circulatory hemodynamics to adjust. Safety is a critical concern; the nurse should always ask for help when needed to prevent injury to the patient and the nurse. The patient on bed rest typically develops orthostatic hypotension; the nurse should check the patient's vital signs before and after she gets up to assess her status and prevent complications.

97 Correct answer—**B**

Sitting up allows maximum lung expansion; taking deep breaths helps build up air behind the mucus and propel it toward the mouth; and holding a pillow against the incision helps to splint it, reducing pain and decreasing the risk of incision rupture. Lying flat on the back or on either side does not allow full lung expansion. Leaning over the overbed table would lessen lung expansion; besides, the overbed table is not an appropriate splint for the incision.

98 Correct answer—**D**

Pain and malaise are subjective symptoms of infection; they must be identified by the patient because the nurse cannot detect them objectively. Pain is caused by pressure on the nerve endings resulting from edema; general malaise is a systemic reaction to infection. Fever, an elevated white blood cell count, swelling, and erythema are objective signs of infection that the nurse can identify by checking vital signs, assessing laboratory test results, and directly observing the wound.

99 Correct answer—A

Sealing the soiled dressing in a plastic bag removes its bacteria, allowing a sterile environment for dressing changes; washing the hands and donning sterile gloves after removing the soiled dressing prevents transferring bacteria from the soiled dressing to the new one. Because the patient is on wound and skin precautions, it is inappropriate to take her to the treatment room, an area used for non-infectious patients. Removing the soiled dressing contaminates the nurse's hands; she should rewash them after removing the soiled dressing and don gloves before applying the sterile one. Removing the soiled dressing contaminates gloves, which then must be changed before applying a sterile dressing. Masks are not required; gowns may be necessary depending on the amount of drainage and the possibility of splashing.

100 Correct answer—B

This wound will heal by secondary intention. This process occurs when a sutured wound is reopened (usually because of infection); granulation on the sides of the open wound fills in the wound cavity. Healing by first intention occurs with an incised, sutured wound; because the edges of the wound are held together, agglutination rather than granulation is involved. Healing by third intention occurs when a wound healing through granulation is sutured to reduce the size of the wound cavity, which is not the case with this patient. Healing by regeneration occurs only with minor injury, such as an abrasion.

Selected references

Books

Alspach, J. *Core Curriculum for Critical Care Nursing,* 4th ed. Philadelphia: W.B. Saunders Co., 1991.

Ayres, S., et al. *Care of the Critically Ill,* 3rd ed. Chicago: Year Book Medical Pubs., 1988.

Bates, B. *A Guide to Physical Examination and History Taking,* 5th ed. Philadelphia: J.B. Lippincott Co., 1989.

Besser, G., et al. *Clinical Endocrinology: An Illustrated Text.* Philadelphia: J.B. Lippincott Co., 1987.

Bluestone, C., and Klein, J. *Otitis Media in Infants and Children.* Philadelphia: W.B. Saunders Co., 1988.

Bork, K., and Brauninger, W. *Diagnosis and Treatment of Skin Diseases.* Philadelphia: W.B. Saunders Co., 1988.

Bradley, J., and Edinberg, M. *Communication in the Nursing Context,* 3rd ed. East Norwalk, Conn.: Appleton & Lange, 1990.

Brunner, L., and Suddarth, D. *The Lippincott Manual of Nursing Practice,* 6th ed. Philadelphia: J.B. Lippincott Co., 1988.

Brunner, L., and Suddarth, D. *Textbook of Medical-Surgical Nursing,* 6th ed. Philadelphia: J.B. Lippincott Co., 1988.

Burtis, G., et al. *Applied Nutrition and Diet Therapy.* Philadelphia: W.B. Saunders Co., 1988.

Burton, G., and Hodgkin, J. *Respiratory Care—A Guide to Clinical Practice,* 3rd ed. Philadelphia: J.B. Lippincott Co., 1991.

Carpenito, L. *Nursing Diagnosis: Application to Clinical Practice,* 3rd ed. Philadelphia: J.B. Lippincott Co., 1989.

Clark, J., et al. *Pharmacological Basics of Nursing Practice,* 3rd ed. St. Louis: Mosby-Year Book, Inc., 1990.

Corbett, J. *Laboratory Test and Diagnostic Procedures with Nursing Diagnoses,* 2nd ed. East Norwalk, Conn.: Appleton & Lange, 1987.

DeWeese, D., et al. *Otolaryngology: Head and Neck Surgery,* 7th ed. St. Louis: C.V Mosby Co., 1988.

Dudek, S. *Nutrition Handbook for Nursing Practice.* Philadelphia: J.B. Lippincott Co., 1987.

Eliopoulos, C. *Gerontological Nursing,* 2nd ed. Philadlephia: J.B. Lippincott Co., 1987.

Fischbach, F. *Manual of Laboratory Diagnostic Tests,* 3rd ed. Philadelphia: J.B. Lippincott Co., 1988.

Gordon, M. *Manual of Nursing Diagnosis 1991-92.* St. Louis: Mosby-Year Book, 1991.

Guyton, A. *Human Physiology and Mechanisms of Disease,* 4th ed. Philadelphia: W.B. Saunders Co., 1987.

Holloway, N. *Nursing the Critically Ill Adult: Applying Nursing Diagnoses,* 3rd ed. Reading, Mass.: Addison-Wesley Publishing Co., 1988.

Holman, S. *Essentials of Nutrition for the Health Professions.* Philadelphia: J.B. Lippincott Co., 1987.

Iyer, P., et al. *Nursing Process and Nursing Diagnosis,* 2nd ed. Philadelphia: W.B. Saunders Co., 1991.

Kee, J. *Handbook of Laboratory and Diagnostic Tests with Nursing Implications,* 3rd ed. East Norwalk, Conn.: Appleton & Lange, 1991.

Kinney, J., and Owen, O. *Nutrition and Metabolism in Patient Care.* Philadelphia: W.B. Saunders Co., 1988.

Lewis, S., and Collier, I. *Medical Surgical Nursing: Assessment and Management of Clinical Problems,* 2nd ed. St. Louis: C.V. Mosby Co., 1987.

Luckmann, J., and Sorensen, K. *Medical-Surgical Nursing: A Psychophysiologic Approach,* 3rd ed. Philadelphia: W.B. Saunders Co., 1987.

Mathewson-Kuhn, M. *Pharmacotherapeutics: A Nursing Process Approach,* 2nd ed. Philadelphia: F.A. Davis Co., 1990.

McKenry, L., and Salerno, E. *Mosby's Pharmacology in Nursing,* 17th ed. St. Louis: C.V. Mosby Co., 1989.

Metheny, N., ed. *Fluid and Electrolyte Balance: Nursing Considerations.* Philadelphia: J.B. Lippincott Co., 1987.

Mott, Sandra, et al. *Nursing Care of Children and Families,* 2nd ed. Reading, Mass.: Addison-Wesley Publishing Co., 1990.

Murray, R., et al. *Psychiatric-Mental Health Nursing,* 3rd ed. East Norwalk, Conn.: Appleton & Lange, 1987.

Patrick, M., et al. *Medical-Surgical Nursing: Pathophysiological Concepts,* 2nd ed. Philadelphia: J.B. Lippincott Co., 1991.

Perry, A., and Potter, P. *Basic Nursing Theory and Practice,* 2nd ed. St. Louis: Mosby-Year Book, Inc., 1991.

Phipps, W., et al. *Medical-Surgical Nursing: Concepts and Clinical Practice,* 4th ed. St. Louis: Mosby-Year Book, Inc., 1991.

Plumer, A., and Lawrence, B. *Principles and Practice of Intravenous Therapy,* 4th ed. Boston: Little, Brown & Co., 1987.

Robinson, C. *Normal and Therapeutic Nutrition,* 17th ed. (rev.). New York: Macmillian Publishing Co., 1990.

Rowe, J., and Beodine, R. *Geriatric Medicine,* 2nd ed. Boston: Little, Brown & Co., 1988.

Seidel, H., et al. *Mosby's Guide to Physical Examination.* St. Louis: C.V. Mosby Co., 1987.

Shapiro, B., et al. *Clinical Application of Respiratory Care,* 4th ed. St. Louis: Mosby-Year Book, 1991.

Skidmore-Roth, L. *Mosby's 1991 Nursing Drug Reference.* St. Louis: Mosby-Year Book, Inc., 1991.

Spencer, R., et al. *Clinical Pharmacology and Nursing Management,* 3rd ed. Philadelphia: J.B. Lippincott Co., 1989.

Thompson, J., et al. *Mosby's Manual of Clinical Nursing,* 2nd ed. St. Louis: C.V. Mosby Co., 1989.

Whaley, L., and Wong, D. *Essentials of Pediatric Nursing,* 3rd ed. St. Louis: C.V. Mosby Company, 1989.

Periodicals

Bayley, E., and Smith, G. "The Three Degrees of Burn Care," *Nursing87* 17(3):34-42, 1987.

Beisecker, A., et al. "Patients' Perspectives of the Role of Care Providers in Amyotrophic Lateral Sclerosis," *Archives of Neurology* 45(5): 553-556, May 1988.

Birch, E., and Stager, D. "Prevalence of Good Visual Acuity Following Surgery for Congenital Unilateral Cataract," *Archives of Ophthalmology* 106(1):40-43, January 1988.

Brune, M., et al. "Iron Absorption: No Intestinal Adaptation to a High-Phytate Diet," *The American Journal of Clinical Nutrition* 49(3):542-45, March 1989.

Busse, J., and Materson, B. "Geriatric Hypertension: The Growing Use of Calcium-Channel Blockers," *Geriatrics* 43(2):51-58, February 1988.

Callahan, M., and Bradley, D. "Why You Should Teach Your Diabetic Patients to Chart," *Nursing88* 18(3):48-49, March 1988.

Coleman, D., et al. "A Worse-Case Guide for Any Case of Psoriasis," *RN* 51(3):39-43, March 1988.

Cox, J., and Jacobs, C. "Laser-Assisted Angioplasty," *AORN Journal* 46(5):57-61, November 1987.

Cunningham, J., et al. "Measured and Predicted Calorie Requirements of Adults During Recovery from Severe Burn Trauma," *American Journal of Clinical Nutrition* 49(3):404-08, March 1989.

Daeschner, S. "Action Stat: Pulmonary Embolism," *Nursing88* 18(9):33, September 1988.

Donehower, M. "Malignant Complications of AIDS," *Oncology Nursing Forum* 14(1): 57-63, 1987.

Eisenberger, M., et al. "How Effective is Cytotoxic Chemotherapy for Disseminated Prostatic Carcinoma?" *Oncology* 1(4):59-71, June 1987.

Fleming, C. "Trace Element Metabolism in Adult Patients Requiring Total Parenteral Nutrition," *American Journal of Clinical Nutrition* 49(3):573-79, March 1989.

Gerdes, L. "Recognizing the Multisystemic Effects of Embolism," *Nursing87* 17(12):34-41, December 1987.

Guzek, J., et al. "Risk Factors for Intraoperative Complications in 1000 Extracapsular Cataract Cases," *Opthalmology* 94(5):461-466, May 1987.

Hemry, M. "Cardiac Rehab: Still Running? or Standing Still?" *AJN* 88(9):1196-1201, September 1988.

Holmes, P. "Sexuality: New Treatments for Impotence," *Nursing Times* 83(34):42-43, 1987.

Hurxthal, K. "Quick! Teach This Patient About Insulin," *American Journal of Nursing* 88(8):1097-1100, August 1988.

Kozinn, S., and Wilson, P. Jr. "Adult Hip Disease and Total Hip Replacement," *Clinical Symposia* 39(5):2-32, 1987.

Krane, R. "Penile Prostheses," *Urological Clinics of North America* 15(1):103-09, February 1988.

Lambert, V., and Lambert, C. "Coping with Rheumatoid Arthritis," *Nursing Clinics of North America* 22(3):551-558, September 1987.

Lowe, B., and Listrom, M. "Management of Stage A Prostate Cancer with a High Probability of Progression," *The Journal of Urology* 140(6):1345-47, December 1988.

Ludwick, R. "Breast Examination in the Older Adult," *Cancer Nursing* 11(2):99-102, April 1988.

Marecki, M. "Chlamydia Trachomatis: A Developing Perinatal Problem," *Journal of Perinatal and Neonatal Nursing* 1(4):1-11, April 1988.

Mayer, D. "Diagnosis and Management of Intestinal Obstruction in Individuals with Cancer," *Nurse Practitioner* 11(2):36-41, February 1986.

Meredith, T., and Acierno, L. "Pulmonary Complications of Acquired Immunodeficiency Syndrome," *Heart & Lung* 17(2):173-78, March 1988.

McCrae, J., and Hall, N. "Current Practices for Home Enteral Nutrition," *Journal of the American Dietetic Association* 89(2):233-40, February 1989.

McLean, A., et al. "Prevalence of Hepatitis B Serologic Markers in Community Hospital Personnel," *American Journal of Public Health* 77(8): 998-999, August 1987.

Miller, R., and Evans, W. "Nurse and Patient: Allies Preventing Amputation," *RN* 51(7):38-44, July 1988.

Morris, L., et al. "Nursing the Patient in Traction," *RN* 51(1):26-31, January 1988.

Patras, A., et al. "Managing GI Bleeding: It Takes a Two-Tract Mind," *Nursing88* 18(4): 68-74, April 1988.

"Position of the American Dietetic Association: Vegetarian Diets-A Technical Support Paper," *Journal of the American Dietetic Association* 88(3):352-55, March 1988.

Powers, M. "Diabetes Nutritional Management," in *Handbook of Diabetes Nutritional Management*. Edited by Powers, M. Rockville, Md.: Aspen Systems Corp., 1987.

Ritchey, A. "Iron Deficiency in Children," *Postgraduate Medicine* 82(2):59-69.

Rossini, A., et al. "Speculation on the Etiology of Diabetes Mellitus: Tumbler Hypothesis," *Diabetes* 37(3):257-61, March 1988.

Schoenfield, L., et al. "Gallstones," *Clinical Symposia, CIBA-GEIGY* 40(2):1-88, 1988.

Smith, C. "Assessing Bowel Sounds," *Nursing88* 18(2):42-43, February 1988.

Smith, C. "Assessing Chest Pain Quickly and Accurately," *Nursing88* 18(5):52-59, May 1988.

Stevens, S., and Becker, K. "A Simple, Step-by-Step Approach to Neurologic Assessment (Part 1)," *Nursing88* 18(9):53-61, September 1988.

Stevens, S., and Becker, K. "How to Perform Picture-Perfect Respiratory Assessment," *Nursing88* 18(1):57-63, January 1988.

Williams, A., et al. "HIV Infection in Intravenous Drug Abusers," *Image: Journal of Nursing Scholarship* 19(4):179-85, Winter 1987.

Wood, E. "Evaluation of a Hospital-Based Education Program for Patients with Diabetes," *Journal of the American Dietetic Association* 89(3):354-58, March 1989.

York, K. "The Lung and Fluid-Electrolyte and Acid-Base Imbalances," *Nursing Clinics of North America* 22(4):805-14, December 1987.

Index